Youness EL ACHHAB

Type 2 diabetes

Youness EL ACHHAB

Type 2 diabetes

Epidemiology, pathophysiology and genetics

ScienciaScripts

Imprint

Cover image: www.ingimage.com

This book is a translation from the original published under ISBN 978-620-3-44980-8.

Publisher:
Sciencia Scripts
is a trademark of
Dodo Books Indian Ocean Ltd. and OmniScriptum S.R.L publishing group

120 High Road, East Finchley, London, N2 9ED, United Kingdom
Str. Armeneasca 28/1, office 1, Chisinau MD-2012, Republic of Moldova, Europe
Printed at: see last page
ISBN: 978-620-5-74791-9

TYPE 2 DIABETES: EPIDEMIOLOGY, PATHOPHYSIOLOGY AND GENETICS

Youness EL ACHHAB

Contents

General introduction

Type 2 diabetes (T2D) is a major public health problem due to its high and increasing prevalence and its ever-increasing socio-economic impact. As a result, T2DM is currently one of the most worrying diseases in both industrialised and developing countries. Thus, diabetes affects more than 537 million people in the world population and more than 784 million by 2045 (International Diabetes Federation 2021).

The common forms of T2DM are polygenic and multifactorial diseases. The environment, a sedentary lifestyle, poorly balanced nutrition and obesity play an important role in this disease, but these factors are all the more decisive if the subject has a family predisposition to becoming diabetic. Thus, not all obese people are diabetic; the 20-30% who become so are those who carry predisposing genes. Indeed, a good definition of the aetiology of T2DM will produce new therapeutic leads and more individualised interventions and treatments.

In addition, genetics represents an important approach to the prediction of diseases with complex inheritance. Thus, evidence has demonstrated the usefulness of intervention in a population at risk of developing T2DM through genetic information.

The molecular and physiological mechanisms by which T2DM is established are only partially elucidated. The use of the whole genome approach over the last two decades has proven to be an effective means of identifying new pathophysiological pathways involved in metabolic alterations.

This book on T2DM is certainly a book that provides a solid foundation and scientific information in a simple way, so that it can be understood by all readers, thus allowing them to understand and de-dramatise diabetes in its entirety, with its complications, to help in the prevention and monitoring of illnesses associated with diabetic disease, or simply to learn more about a disease that is increasingly permeating our daily lives.

CHAPTER 1

TYPE 2 DIABETES: EPIDEMIOLOGY

1. Diabetes in the Ages

Diabetes is a very old disease (Von Engelhardt 1989). The disease is mentioned in ancient writings of Chinese and Egyptian medicine. Reference is often made to the papyrus dating from 1550 BC and discovered in Luxor by the German Egyptologist Ebers. In the 2ème century AD, Arrested of Cappadocia gives a vivid description of the disease while Galen attributes it to the inability of the kidneys to retain water. At the end of the first millennium AD, Ibn Sinna, better known as Avicenna, described the condition more accurately and noted that it could be complicated by gangrene. The "sweet taste" of urine, already reported in the 7ème century by Chinese and Indian physicians, was rediscovered in 1674 by Thomas Willis, who made the distinction between *diabetes mellitus* and *diabetes* insipidus. èmeIt was in the second half of the 19th century that Claude Bernard described in Paris the essential characteristics of carbohydrate metabolism and the role played by the liver in this (Lefèbvre *et al.* 1996).

In 1869, Paul Langerhans described, for the first time, the presence in the pancreatic gland of small cell clusters known under his name of islets of Langerhans. Work in the 20th century demonstrated that these cells are endocrine in nature and secrete various hormones including insulin and glucagon. The notion that the pancreas manufactures a substance that prevents the onset of diabetes quickly developed. This substance, which was still hypothetical, was named 'insulin' by De Meyer in Brussels before it was even isolated. The name insulin indicates that it originates in the islets described by Langerhans. Shortly after Paulesco's work (Paulesco 1921), Canadian authors reported the isolation of insulin from the pancreas in 1921 and, as early as 1922, the successful treatment with insulin of the first patient with diabetes, the young Leonard Thompson (Lefèbvre 1996).

This brief overview of the history of diabetes does not end here. Clinicians had long observed that some patients with diabetes, especially in children, adolescents and young adults, suffered from a severe form of the disease, which was fatal without insulin treatment. Long known as 'lean', 'consumptive' or 'insulin-dependent' diabetes, this form of the disease, which affects a minority of patients, is now called 'type 1 diabetes'.

In contrast, there are many more patients who also have diabetes but survive for many years without the need for insulin injections. These patients, often older, were said to have "fat", "plethoric" or "mature" diabetes. Today we say "type 2 diabetes".

2. Definition

T2DM is the most common metabolic disease in the world. It accounts for more than 90% of diagnosed diabetes cases and is largely preventable by adopting a healthy lifestyle (Zhang *et al.* 2020; WHO 2020). It usually occurs in people over 40 years of age, who have a family history of diabetes and are overweight. In contrast to type 1 diabetes, T2DM is a complex disease that is usually part of the broader metabolic syndrome. Its aetiology is determined by the interaction of genetic and environmental factors (Geng & Huang 2020). Pathophysiologically, it results from a combination of varying degrees of abnormalities in insulin secretion and action (Galicia-Garcia *et al.* 2020), which accounts for its heterogeneous phenotype.

The chronic hyperglycaemia of diabetes causes significant long-term damage, dysfunction and failure of various organs: kidneys, eyes, nerves, heart and blood vessels, etc.

3. Diagnosis

According to the "Standards of Medical Care in Diabetes" published by the American Diabetes Association (ADA 2022) and the World Health Organization (WHO 2020) guidelines, diabetes can be diagnosed on the basis of plasma glucose concentration - either fasting plasma glucose (FPG) or two-hour plasma glucose in a 75 g oral glucose tolerance test (OGTT) - or on the basis of glycated haemoglobin A1c (HbA1c) concentration (Tab. 1).

Prediabetes is a state of intermediate hyperglycaemia in which glycaemic indices such as blood glucose and HbA1c are above the threshold considered normal but below the diagnostic criteria for diabetes. This state constitutes a high risk for the development of diabetes and complications associated with loss of glycaemic control (Echouffo-Tcheugui & Selvin 2021).

Table 1. Diagnosis of diabetes: Reference values (ADA 2022 & WHO 2020)

	FPG	**OGTT, 2h**	**HbA1c**
Prediabetes			
ADA	100-125 mg/dL	140-199 mg/dL	5,7-6,4 %
WHO	110-125 mg/dL	-	NR
Diabetes			
ADA	≥ 126 mg/dL	≥ 200 mg/dL	≥ 6,5 %
WHO	≥ 126 mg/dL	≥ 200 mg/dL	≥ 6,5 %

FPG, fasting plasma glucose; HbA1c, glycated hemoglobin A1c; OGTT, oral glucose tolerance test; ADA, American Diabetes Association; WHO, World Health Organization; NR, not recommended.

The diagnosis of type 2 diabetes is usually made on the basis of a screening blood glucose test in an android overweight individual over 35 years of age, with elements of the metabolic syndrome reflecting insulin resistance (high waist circumference, hypertension, dyslipaemia), and a family and/or obstetric history (gestational diabetes or neonatal macrosomia) for women. Family history is present in the majority of cases. First-degree relatives of a person with type 2 diabetes have a 20% lifetime risk of developing a glycome disorder (Rigalleau *et al.* 2020).

4. Prevalence

The prevalence and incidence of T2DM is rapidly increasing in both industrialised and developing countries (Tinajero & Malik 2021). In the year 2021, the International Diabetes Federation (IDF) estimates that 537 million of the world's population aged 20-79 years are diabetics (IDF 2021). In its latest global estimate, the IDF stated that the number of people with diabetes worldwide will increase from 634 million in 2030 to 784 million in the year 2045 (IDF 2021) (Fig. 1). According to the same IDF report, more than 3 in 4 adults with diabetes live in low- and middle-income countries.

More recently, the largest percentage increases in age-standardised prevalence of T2DM have occurred in the Middle East and North Africa (MENA) and South Asia (Tinajero & Malik 2021); regions that have undergone rapid epidemiological transitions in recent decades such as urbanisation, declining nutritional quality and increasing sedentary behaviour.

The largest percentage increases in T2DM prevalence will be in African countries (134%) and the MENA region (87%) (IDF 2021).

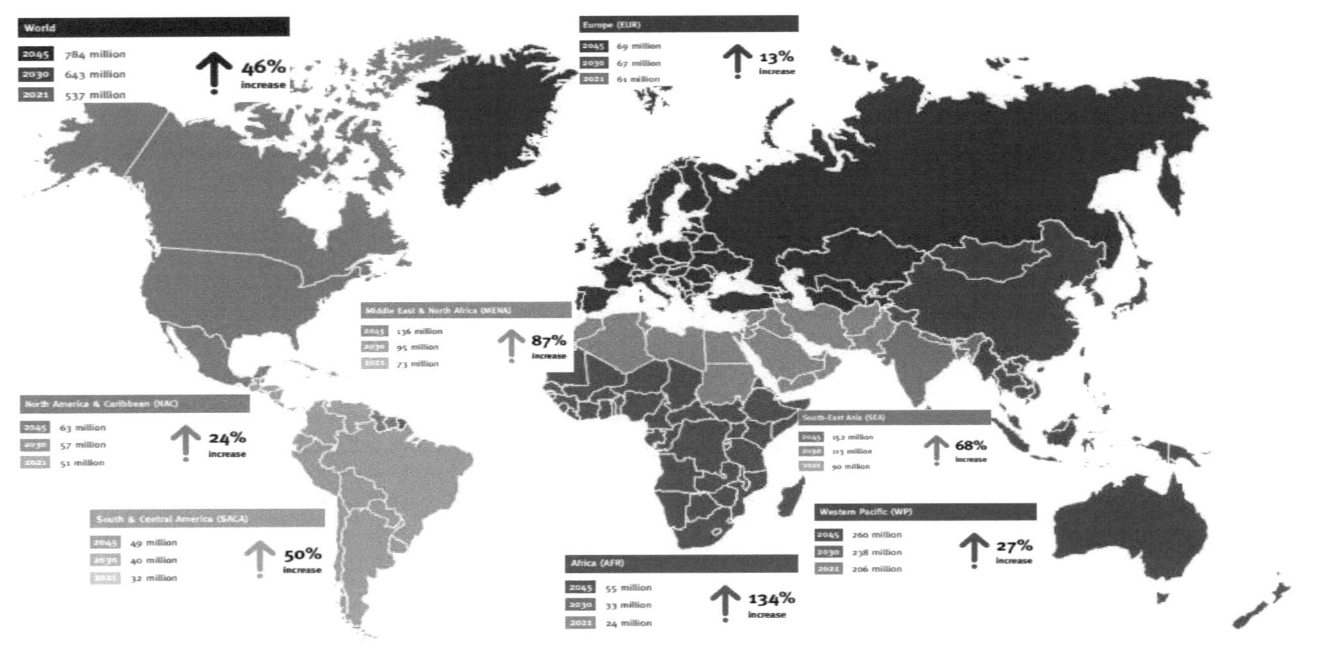

Figure 1: Distribution of diabetics (20-79 years) in millions in the world in 2021 and forecasts for the year 2030 and 2045 with expected percentage change. *Adapted from the International Diabetes Federation (2021)*

5. Risk factors

T2DM is a complex disease characterised by a multitude of risk factors, some of which are modifiable (Fig. 2). There is usually a strong genetic component (predisposing terrain) on top of which are environmental factors, some of which may already exert their effects during intrauterine life, through epigenetic mechanisms (Fernandez-Twinn *et al.* 2019).

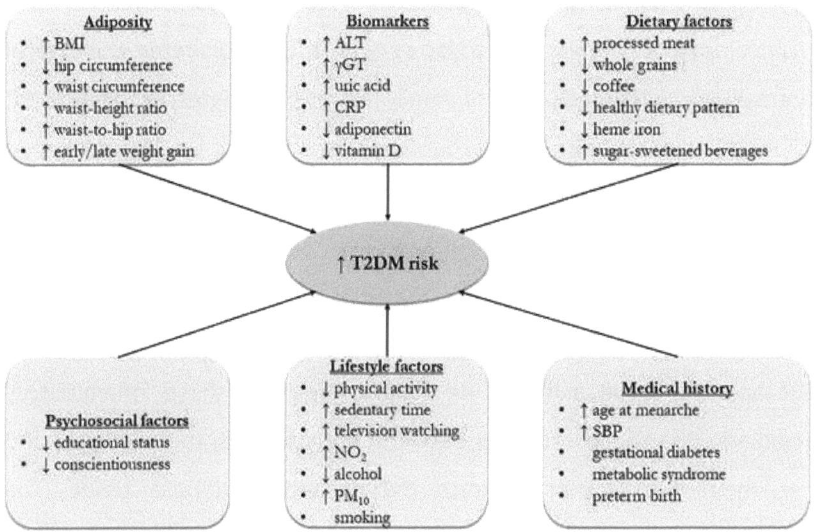

Figure 2: Risk factors for T2D with evidence-based arguments. Adapted from (Bellou *et al.* 2018).

Overweight, abdominal obesity and physical inactivity are the most important risk factors for the development of T2DM (Carbone *et al.* 2019; Anderson &

Durstine 2019). Thus, the dramatic increase in the proportion of diabetics has occurred in settings that have rapidly adopted a Western-style lifestyle. These include marked changes in behaviour, such as the abandonment of physical exercise and the consumption of high-energy foods and drinks. Within a few years, the majority of the population became obese (Blüher 2019). Regular physical activity (at least 30 min per day 5 times per week) reduces the risk of developing T2D (Burr *et al.* 2010). In the T2DM patient, this approach contributes to significantly improve not only glycaemic control but also that of other cardiovascular risk factors (Bassuk & Manson 2005; Kemps *et al.* 2019).

Age, impaired glucose tolerance, a history of gestational diabetes, cholesterol abnormalities, high blood pressure, family history of diabetes and a history of cardiovascular disease are also recognised as risk factors for T2D (Alberti et al. 2007).

Epidemiological studies have established an association between inflammatory biomarkers and the occurrence of T2D and complications (Lontchi-Yimagou *et al.* 2013; Cruz *et al.* 2013; Burhans *et al.* 2018). Adipose tissue appears to be a major site of production of these inflammatory biomarkers, due to the crosstalk between adipose cells, macrophages and other immune cells that infiltrate the expanding adipose tissue. The inflammatory response probably contributes to the development of T2DM by inducing insulin resistance, and is in turn intensified in the presence of hyperglycaemia to promote long-term complications of diabetes. Targeting inflammatory pathways could potentially be part of strategies to prevent and control diabetes and associated complications (Donath 2014).

6. Complications

The severity of diabetes is mainly due to long-term complications that lead to disability, handicap and reduced quality of life. Since T2DM can remain undetected for a long time, it is not uncommon for diabetes to be diagnosed in the face of one of these complications. The complications of diabetes can be separated into two broad categories: macrovascular complications (coronary artery disease, cerebrovascular disease and peripheral vascular disease) and microvascular complications (retinopathy, nephropathy, neuropathy and foot problems).

Prospective epidemiological studies have shown that chronic hyperglycaemia plays an important role in the pathogenesis of microvascular and macrovascular complications in diabetes (Chawla *et al.* 2016; Beckman & Creager 2016; Faselis *et al.* 2020). Four main hypotheses have been put forward to explain how hyperglycaemia is able to generate these complications (Brownlee 2005). These four hypotheses are: increased flux in the polyol pathway, increased production of advanced glycation endproducts (AGEs), signal transduction through activation of protein kinase C (PKC) and increased production of hexosamines. A mechanism combining these hypotheses has been suggested (Brownlee 2005).

In an observational study, involving 28 countries in Asia, Africa, South America and Europe, complications related to T2DM are very common, with half of the patients having microvascular complications and 27% with macrovascular complications (Litwak *et al.* 2013).

References

Alberti, K. G. M. M., Zimmet, P., & Shaw, J. (2007). International Diabetes Federation: a consensus on Type 2 diabetes prevention. Diabetic Medicine, 24(5), 451-463.

American Diabetes Association Professional Practice Committee, & American Diabetes Association Professional Practice Committee (2022). 2. Classification and diagnosis of diabetes: standards of medical care in diabetes-2022. Diabetes Care, 45(Sup_1), S17-S38.

Anderson, E., & Durstine, J. L. (2019). Physical activity, exercise, and chronic diseases: A brief review. *Sports Medicine and Health Science*, 1(1), 3-10.

Bassuk, S. S., & Manson, J. E. (2005). Epidemiological evidence for the role of physical activity in reducing risk of type 2 diabetes and cardiovascular disease. *Journal of applied physiology*.

Beckman, J. A., & Creager, M. A. (2016). Vascular complications of diabetes. *Circulation research*, *118*(11), 1771-1785.

Bellou, V., Belbasis, L., Tzoulaki, I., & Evangelou, E. (2018). Risk factors for type 2 diabetes mellitus: an exposure-wide umbrella review of meta-analyses. *PloS one*, *13*(3), e0194127.

Blüher, M. (2019). Obesity: global epidemiology and pathogenesis. *Nature Reviews Endocrinology*, 15(5), 288-298.

Brownlee, M. (2005). The pathobiology of diabetic complications: a unifying mechanism. Diabetes, 54(6), 1615-1625.

Burhans, M. S., Hagman, D. K., Kuzma, J. N., Schmidt, K. A., & Kratz, M. (2018). Contribution of adipose tissue inflammation to the development of type 2 diabetes mellitus. Comprehensive Physiology, 9(1), 1.

Burr, J. F., Rowan, C. P., Jamnik, V. K., & Riddell, M. C. (2010). The role of physical activity in type 2 diabetes prevention: physiological and practical perspectives. The Physician and sportsmedicine, 38(1), 72-82.

Carbone, S., Del Buono, M. G., Ozemek, C., & Lavie, C. J. (2019). Obesity, risk of diabetes and role of physical activity, exercise training and cardiorespiratory fitness. *Progress in cardiovascular diseases*, 62(4), 327-333.

Chawla, A., Chawla, R., & Jaggi, S. (2016). Microvasular and macrovascular complications in diabetes mellitus: distinct or continuum?" *Indian journal of endocrinology and metabolism*, 20(4), 546.

Cruz, N. G., Sousa, L. P., Sousa, M. O., Pietrani, N. T., Fernandes, A. P., & Gomes, K. B. (2013). The linkage between inflammation and Type 2 diabetes mellitus. Diabetes research and clinical practice, 99(2), 85-92.

Donath, M. Y. (2014). Targeting inflammation in the treatment of type 2 diabetes: time to start. *Nature reviews Drug discovery*, *13*(6), 465-476.

Echouffo-Tcheugui, J. B., & Selvin, E. (2021). Prediabetes and what it means: the epidemiological evidence. Annual Review of Public Health, 42, 59-77.

Faselis, C., Katsimardou, A., Imprialos, K., Deligkaris, P., Kallistratos, M., & Dimitriadis, K. (2020). Microvascular complications of type 2 diabetes mellitus. Current vascular pharmacology, 18(2), 117-124.

Fernandez-Twinn, D. S., Hjort, L., Novakovic, B., Ozanne, S. E., & Saffery, R. (2019). Intrauterine programming of obesity and type 2 diabetes. Diabetologia, 62(10), 1789-1801.

Geng, T., & Huang, T. (2020). Gene-environment interactions and type 2 diabetes. Asia Pacific Journal of Clinical Nutrition, 29(2), 220-226.

Galicia-Garcia, U., Benito-Vicente, A., Jebari, S., Larrea-Sebal, A., Siddiqi, H., Uribe, K. B., ... & Martín, C. (2020). Pathophysiology of type 2 diabetes mellitus. International journal of molecular sciences, 21(17), 6275.

International Diabetes Federation (2021). IDF diabetes atlas. 10th ed. Brussels: International Diabetes Federation.

Kemps, H., Kränkel, N., Dörr, M., Moholdt, T., Wilhelm, M., Paneni, F., ... & Guazzi, M. (2019). Exercise training for patients with type 2 diabetes and cardiovascular disease: What to pursue and how to do it. A Position Paper of the European Association of Preventive Cardiology (EAPC). European Journal of Preventive Cardiology, 26(7), 709-727.

Litwak, L., Goh, S. Y., Hussein, Z., Malek, R., Prusty, V., & Khamseh, M. E. (2013). Prevalence of diabetes complications in people with type 2 diabetes mellitus and its association with baseline characteristics in the multinational A1chieve study. Diabetology & metabolic syndrome, 5(1), 1-10.

Lontchi-Yimagou, E., Sobngwi, E., Matsha, T. E., & Kengne, A. P. (2013). Diabetes mellitus and inflammation. *Current diabetes reports*, *13*(3), 435-444.

Rigalleau V., Monlun M., Foussard N., Blanco L., Mohammedi K. (2020). Diagnosis of diabetes. EMC - AKOS (Traité de Médecine);24(1):1-7.

Tinajero, M. G., & Malik, V. S. (2021). An update on the epidemiology of type 2 diabetes: a global perspective. Endocrinology and Metabolism Clinics, 50(3), 337-355.

World Health Organization (2020). Diagnosis and management of type 2 diabetes (HEARTS-D). Geneva; (WHO/UCN/NCD/20.1).

Zhang, Y., Pan, X. F., Chen, J., Xia, L., Cao, A., Zhang, Y., ... & Pan, A. (2020). Combined lifestyle factors and risk of incident type 2 diabetes and prognosis among individuals with type 2 diabetes: a systematic review and meta-analysis of prospective cohort studies. *Diabetologia*, *63*(1), 21-33.

CHAPTER 2

TYPE 2 DIABETES: PHYSIOLOGY AND PATHOPHYSIOLOGY

T2DM is characterised by two metabolic abnormalities, the relative importance of which varies from one form to another: a deficit in insulin secretion or insulinopenia, and a decrease in the sensitivity to insulin of the target tissues, mainly muscle, liver and adipose tissue, also known as insulin resistance.

1. Insulin secretion and signalling pathway

When blood glucose levels rise, glucose entry into pancreaticβ cells occurs through the insulin-independent glucose transporter GLUT2, which is followed by phosphorylation of glucose by glucokinases (Fig. 3). This phosphorylation helpsβ cells to detect fluctuating glucose levels and respond to extracellular changes. Intracellular glucose degradation or glycolysis causes the production of ATP and thereby induces the closure of ATP-dependent potassium channels. This results in membrane depolarisation of the pancreaticβ cells, which causes the opening of calcium-dependent channels. The massive influx of calcium promotes the translocation of insulin-secreting vesicles to the cytoplasmic membrane and the exocytosis of insulin. This corresponds to the first phase of insulin secretion which takes place within 5 minutes of glucose loading. A second, slower and more sustained phase occurs thereafter and corresponds to the replenishment of preformed secretory granules (Fig. 4) (Aizawa & Komatsu 2005).

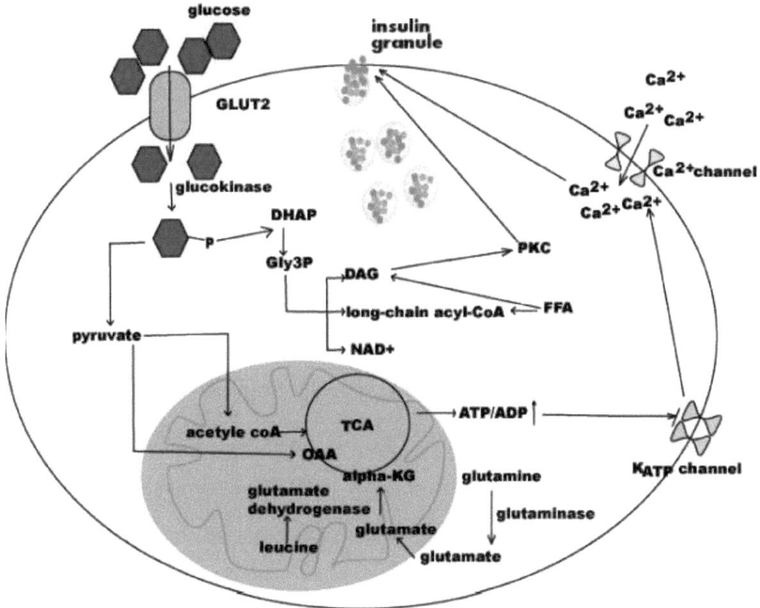

Figure 3: Mechanisms of insulin secretion in the pancreatic β cell. From (Fu *et al.* 2013).

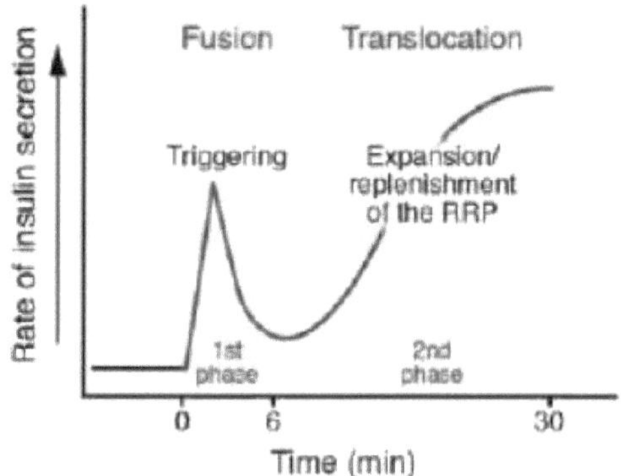

Figure 4: Representation of glucose-stimulated biphasic insulin secretion. Adapted from (Aizawa & Komatsu 2005).

The target tissues of insulin, which are the liver, muscle and adipose tissue, will be affected (Fig. 5). At the level of the adipocyte, insulin will promote glucose storage, inhibiting lipolysis genes and activating lipogenesis genes (Petersen & Shulman 2018). In muscle, it will promote glucose uptake, glycogen synthesis and activation of key enzymes in the glycogenogenesis cascade (Björnholm & Zierath 2005; Petersen & Shulman 2018). In the liver, it will inhibit glycogenolysis and thus hepatic glucose production (Petersen & Shulman 2018). Thus, the consequence of these phenomena is the uptake of glucose in the target tissues and the establishment of normal blood glucose levels.

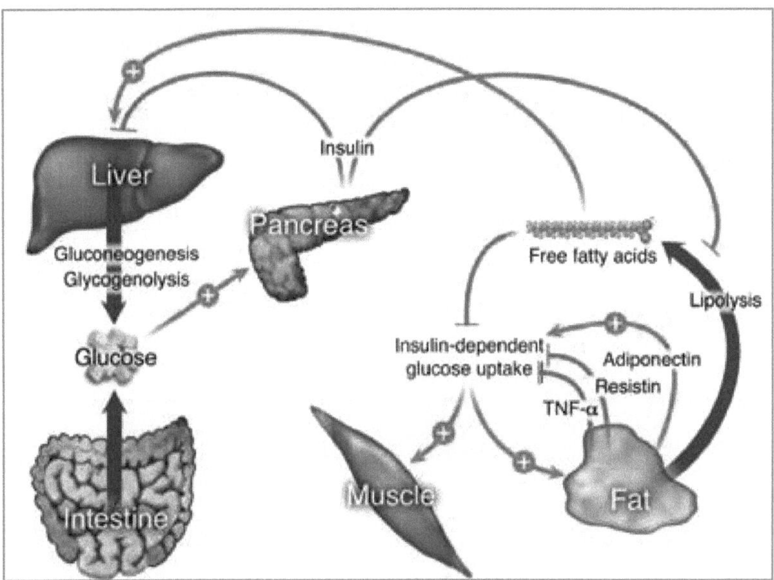

Figure 5: Interaction between the different organs involved in the maintenance of carbohydrate and lipid homeostasis (Jahandideh & Wu 2022).

The insulin receptor belongs to the family of growth factor receptors that have tyrosine kinase activity in their intracellular domain. It is a four-subunit protein belonging to the receptor tyrosine kinase family (Chang *et al.* 2004). The receptor consists of two extracellular α-subunits that bind insulin and inhibit the tyrosine kinase activity of the two β-subunits. Insulin binding to the α-subunits lifts the inhibition of the β-subunits and leads to their autophosphorylation and thus to an increase in their tyrosine kinase activity (Tokarz *et al.* 2018) (Fig. 6). This phase is followed by the mobilisation of several intracellular substrates that are phosphorylated such as the IRS (Insulin Receptor Substrate 1-4) family. The phosphorylated tyrosines of these substrates act as anchor sites for proteins that contain SH2 (Src-homology-2) domains and activate a series of signalling pathways including Phosphatidyl

Inositol 3 (PI3) Kinase and MAP Kinase (Mitogen Activated Protein). The PI3 kinase pathway plays a key role in glucose transport via the activation of Akt/PKB kinase, which stimulates the membrane translocation of GLUT4 glucose transporters (Fu et al. 2013, Tokarz et al. 2018). The MAP kinase pathway activates gene expression and proliferation. The PI3 kinase/PKB and MAP kinase pathways are interconnected and participate in each other's activation (Capeau 2003).

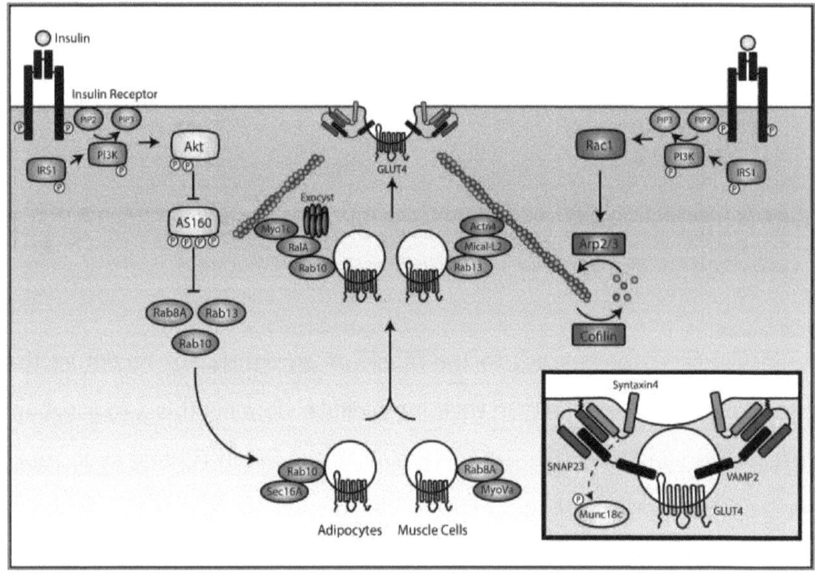

Figure 6: Transduction signals involved in insulin action in muscle and fat cells. From (Tokarz *et al.* 2018).

2. Alterations in insulin secretion

Alterations in insulin secretion are the common denominator of all forms of diabetes (Guillausseau & Laloi-Michelin 2003). They appear early in the history of T2DM. These alterations are classified under five headings, grouped under the term of insular dysfunction: pulsatility abnormalities, kinetic abnormalities, qualitative abnormalities, quantitative abnormalities and evolutionary abnormalities.

In non-diabetics, insulin is secreted in the basal state in a pulsatile mode (Bergsten 2000). In T2DM, there is a decrease or disappearance of the rapid oscillatory secretion of insulin (Rutter *et al.* 2015). A disappearance of the early phase of insulin secretion in response to glucose is common in chronic hyperglycaemia (Temple *et al.* 1992). The proportion of insulin secreted as pro-insulin, which is normally very low in normal subjects, increases with the severity of diabetes, which is generally attributed to insufficient maturation of the secretory process due to hyperstimulation of ß-cells by hyperglycaemia (Steiner 2000). Finally, insulin secretion in patients with T2DM is characterised by its progressive reduction over time and by its programmed depletion (Fig. 7) (Permutt *et al.* 2005).

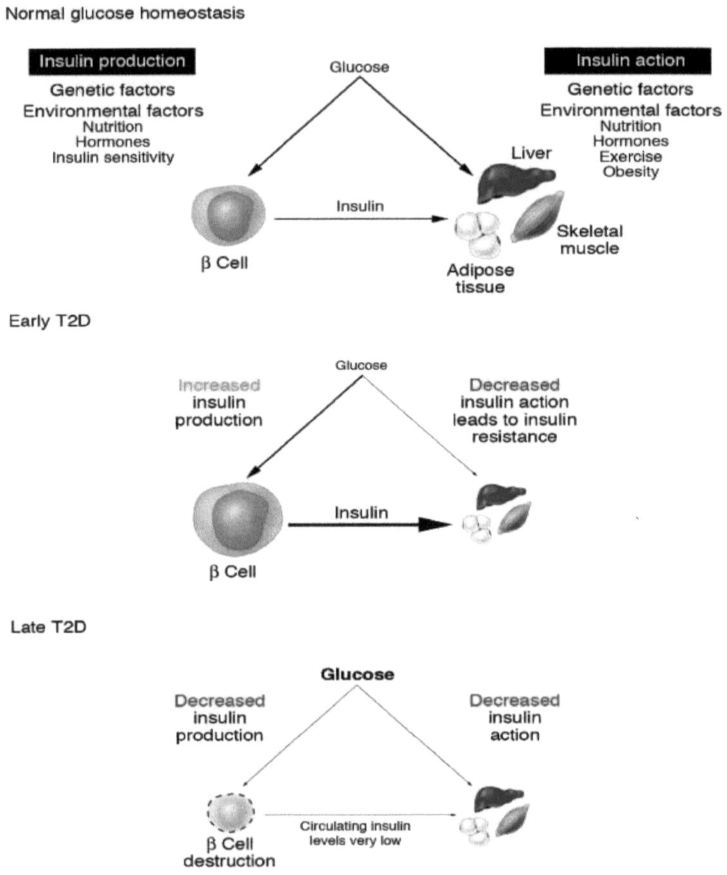

Figure 7: Type 2 diabetes: the result of an imbalance between the production of insulin by pancreatic β-cells and its action on target tissues such as liver, muscle and adipose tissue. According to (Permutt *et al.* 2005).

3. Alterations in insulin sensitivity and pancreatic β-cell failure

The vast majority of type 2 diabetic patients have varying degrees of resistance to insulin action and pancreatic β-cell failure (Marchetti *et al.* 2008; Muoio & Newgard 2008). This resistance occurs in the three main target tissues of the hormone: liver, skeletal muscle and adipose tissue. In practice, it is manifested by an increase in hepatic glucose production (mainly from gluconeogenesis), a decrease in muscle glucose uptake (which is compensated for by hyperglycaemia) and exaggerated lipolysis with an increase in plasma free fatty acid levels (Campbell & Newgard 2021). Insulin resistance, induced by hyperglycaemia, provides a persistent stimulus for pancreaticβ cells to increase secretion to meet the insulin requirements of target tissues (Fig. 7). Indeed, Kahn *et al* (1993) demonstrated that a 50% decrease in insulin sensitivity results in a doubling in the secretion ofβ cells to maintain carbohydrate homeostasis. As a result, theβ cells gradually fail to maintain this high rate of insulin secretion and, with increasing hyperglycaemia, insulin levels are reduced. In another study, insulin secretion capacity is reduced to 50% in glucose intolerant subjects and reaches 15% in T2DM subjects (Buchanan 2003).

3.1. Insulin resistance in adipose tissue

Adipose tissue is a metabolically dynamic tissue capable of synthesising a wide range of biologically active compounds that regulate metabolic homeostasis (Coelho *et al.* 2013). In addition, it participates in a wide range of biological processes involving, among others, immunity, coagulation, angiogenesis, fibrinolysis, reproduction, control of vascular tone, regulation of appetite, weight homeostasis and glucose and lipid metabolism (Rosen & Spiegelman 2006).

Adipose tissue produces a variety of bioactive peptides, known as "adipokines", which are involved in different ways in carbohydrate homeostasis (Guerre-Millo 2004). These are, in particular, TNF-α and IL-6 (Interleukin-6). TNF-α, a multifunctional cytokine, is involved in insulin resistance; it inhibits glucose uptake in the adipocyte by impairing insulin-generated phosphorylation (Fig. 8) (Arner 2003). Studies suggest that IL-6 may be involved in insulin resistance and its complications (Kim 2009). Whatever the mechanisms involved, it is now well documented that cytokines, in particular TNF-α and IL-6, are able to decrease the action of insulin (Krogh-Madsen *et al.* 2006). Adipocytes also secrete leptin and adiponectin, which are considered to be anti-diabetogenic factors through their ability to decrease triglyceride synthesis, stimulate β- oxidation and promote insulin action at the level of target tissues (Muoio & Newgard 2008). In type 2 diabetics, lipotoxicity reduces insulin sensitivity in adipose tissue (Delarue & Magnan 2007). Thus, the mechanism involves PKC dependent phosphorylation of serine/threonine residues of SRIs and its inhibitory consequences (Nguyen *et al.* 2005).

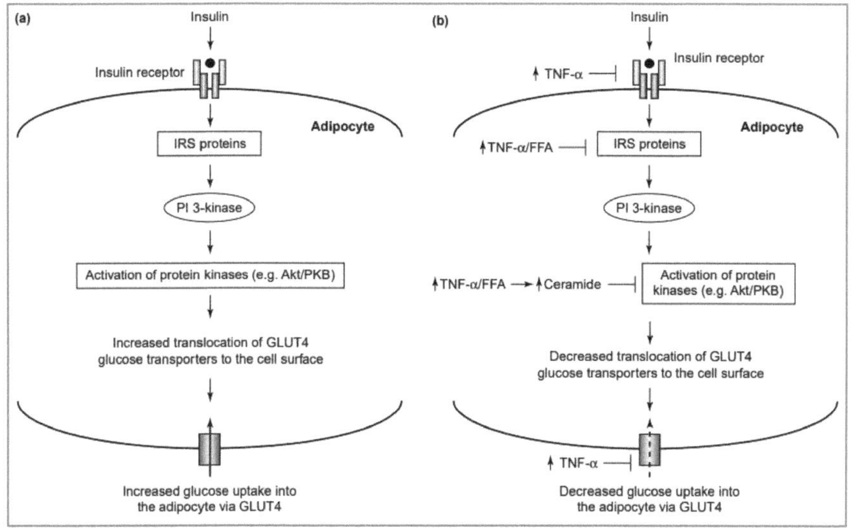

Figure 8: Insulin signalling in the adipocyte. Adapted from (Arner 2003).

(a) *In the normal case, insulin binds to its receptor tyrosine kinase leading to phosphorilation/activation of IRS (insulin receptor substrate) and stimulation of PI3-kinase (phosphatidyl inositol 3-kinase). PI-kinase downstream activates other protein kinases including Akt/PKB. These signalling events result in the influx of glucose into the adipocyte via the translocation of GLUT4 molecules to the cell membrane. The anti-lipolytic effect of insulin is mediated by the activation of PI-kinases which in turn stimulates phosphodiesterase-3, enhancing cAMP metabolism in the adipocyte. This decreases the phosphorrylation of hormone-sensitive lipase, making it less active.* **(b)** *In the insulin-resistant adipocyte, signaling is reduced at different levels, including receptor interaction, tyrosine kinase phosphorylation and activity, IRS protein phosphorylation, downstream activation of Akt/PKB by PI-Kinase and GLUT4 synthesis/translocation to the cell membrane. Certain factors secreted by the adipocyte (e.g. TNF-α (tumor necrosis factor-α) and free fatty acids) appear to play a role in the development of insulin resistance at the adipocyte level through inhibition of insulin signalling.*

3.2. Insulin resistance in the muscle

Glycolysis or glycogen synthesis are two main possible fates of glucose that enters the myocyte upon insulin stimulation. The main pathway of glucose disposal in healthy and type 2 diabetic human muscle is glycogen synthesis (~75%), consistent with the general teleological role of insulin as an energy storage hormone (DeFronzo & Tripathy 2009). The action of muscle insulin is therefore a tightly coordinated relay that serves to promote glucose utilisation and storage (Fig. 9).

In normal subjects, activation of the IRS/PI3-kinase pathway by insulin causes translocation of GLUT4 to the myocyte membrane which in turn promotes glucose entry into the muscle cells and thus glycogen synthesis. In type 2 diabetic subjects, the stimulation of glycogen synthesis is reduced by 50% compared to controls, this being mainly due to a defect in the transport of glucose into skeletal muscle by GLUT4 (Petersen & Shulman 2006).

On the other hand, increased GLA levels in humans cause inhibition of the IRS/PI3K pathway and activation of the PKC pathway (Petersen & Shulman 2018) (Fig. 9). The role of PKC in insulin resistance is well established. Indeed, studies in rats show that activation of PKC-θ by lipid metabolites causes inhibition of IRS tyrosine kinase phosphorylation and a 50% decrease in PI3-K pathway activation (Griffin *et al.* 1999).

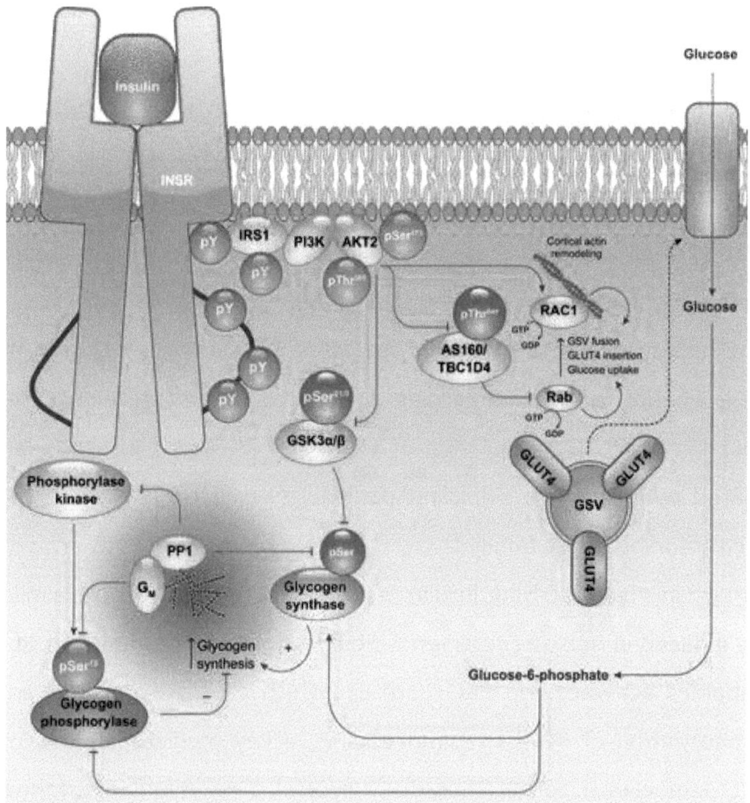

Figure 9: Insulin signalling in muscle. From (Petersen & Shulman 2018).

Insulin receptor activation (INSR) has two major metabolic functions in the skeletal myocyte: glucose uptake and glycogen storage. Insulin stimulation of glucose uptake occurs through translocation of storage vesicles (GSVs) containing GLUT4 to the plasma membrane. The resulting increase in intracellular glucose-6-phosphate production, together with a coordinated dephosphorylation of glycogen metabolic proteins, allows net glycogen synthesis. Green circles and arrows represent activating pathways; red circles and arrows represent inhibitory pathways. GSK3, glycogen synthase kinase 3; PI3K, phosphoinositide-3-kinase; PP1, protein phosphatase 1.

3.3. Insulin resistance in the liver

Liver cells play a key role in glucose storage and production. Insulin stimulates the entry of glucose through GLUT2 into the hepatocytes, which is converted by hepatic glucokinase into glucose-6-phosphate (Fig. 10). Subsequently, the activation of glycogen synthase by insulin promotes glycogen formation and inhibits gluconeogenesis (Leclercq *et al.* 2007).

At the hepatocellular level, insulin regulates the synthesis of three major classes of biological macromolecules: glycogen, lipids and proteins (Petersen & Shulman 2018). The regulation of protein synthesis by insulin is largely mediated by the mTOR signalling pathway (which is an enzyme of the serine/threonine kinase family).

The mechanisms underlying insulin resistance in hepatocytes are similar to those induced in muscle (Petersen & Shulman 2006). Accumulation of lipid metabolites activates the PKC-ε protein which causes a decrease in the phosphorylation of IRS-2 tyrosine residues, a key mediator of the insulin effect (Samuel et al. 2004). Thus, diacylglycerol, a key stimulator of the PKC-ε pathway, potentially mediates this mechanism (Perry et al. 2014).

In type 2 diabetics, the rate of hepatic gluconeogenesis increases and is the immediate cause of the fasting hyperglycaemia that defines this disease (Gastaldelli et al. 2000).

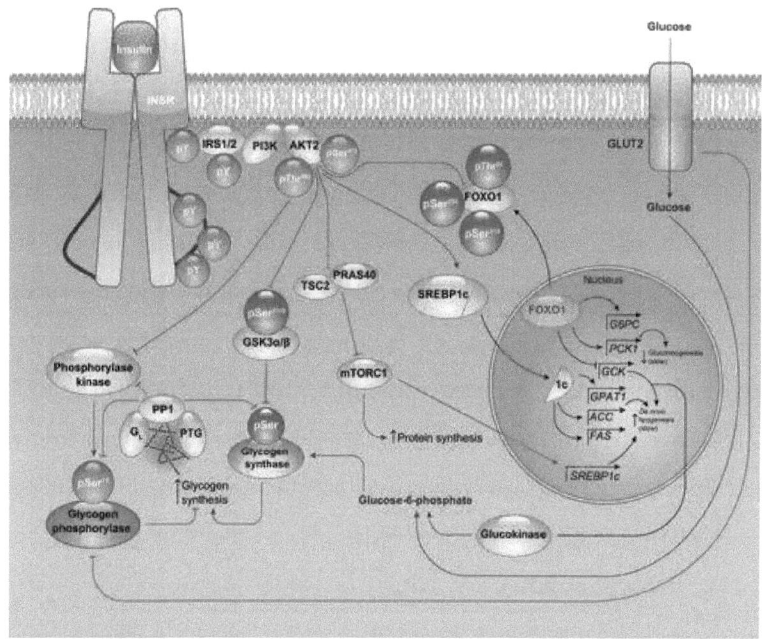

Figure 10: Insulin signalling in the liver. From (Petersen & Shulman 2018).

The action of insulin at the hepatocyte level is primarily via AKT signalling. Rapid effects include activation of the glycogen and protein synthesis machinery. Slower, transcriptionally mediated effects include up-regulation of glucokinase, decrease in gluconeogenic capacity and stimulation of "de novo" lipogenic capacity. Green circles and arrows represent activating pathways; red circles and arrows represent inhibitory pathways. GSK3, glycogen synthase kinase 3; PI3K, phosphoinositide-3-kinase; PP1, protein phosphatase 1; G6PC, glucose-6-phosphatase; PCK1, SREBP1c, sterol regulatory element binding protein 1c.

3.4. Insulin resistance between muscle and liver

Insulin resistance in skeletal muscle usually accompanies insulin resistance at other sites, possibly due to diversion of substrates from insulin-resistant muscle to the liver (Perry *et al.* 2014) (Fig.11).

In insulin-sensitive individuals, insulin stimulates glycogen synthesis in both liver and muscle; however, in individuals with skeletal muscle insulin resistance, insulin fails to promote glycogen synthesis, diverting the substrate to *de novo* lipogenesis. Increased lipid synthesis in patients with muscle insulin resistance thus produces non-alcoholic fatty liver disease (NAFLD), with increased triglycerides and reduced high-density lipoprotein (HDL) export from the liver. However, these defects in muscle insulin signalling can be reversed by a single 45-minute exercise session (Perry *et al.* 2014; Flannery *et al.* 2012; Rabøl *et al.* 2011).

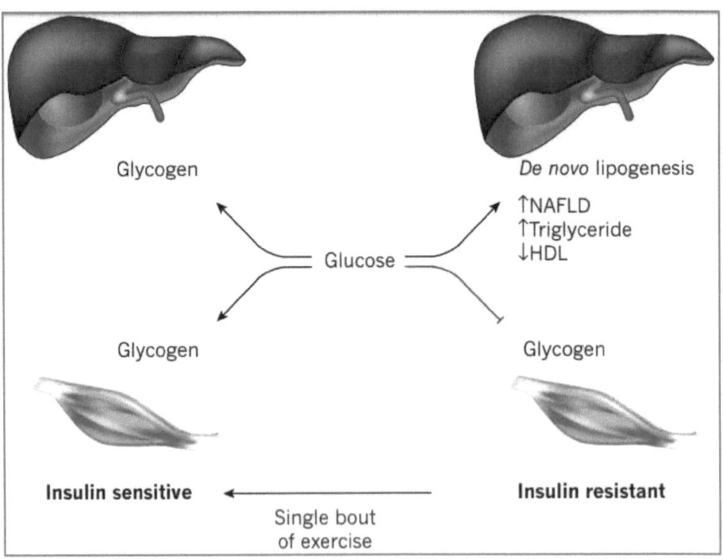

Figure 11: Mechanism by which skeletal muscle insulin resistance contributes to liver insulin resistance. Adapted from (Perry *et al.* 2014).

NAFLD, non-alcoholic fatty liver disease

3.5. Insulin resistance: a link between T2D and obesity

The term 'diabesity' is now used to define the increasing prevalence of diabetes in relation to obesity (Zimmet 2007). Anything that affects body weight represents a greater risk factor for the development of T2DM: high BMI, increased waist circumference, long duration of overweight and/or rapid weight gain are among the main factors promoting insulin resistance, β-cell decompensation and impaired glucose tolerance (Hu *et al.* 2001; Scheen 2000). Conversely, 80% of T2DM subjects are diagnosed as obese. However, triglyceride agglomeration in adipocytes, particularly at the visceral level, contributes to the formation of large insulin-resistant adipocytes resulting in excessive triglyceride lipolysis (Poitout and Robertson 2008). This increases free fatty acids in the circulation causing the aggravation of insulin resistance in muscle and liver. Furthermore, chronic exposure of the pancreas to high concentrations of fatty acids leads to an accumulation of acyl Co-A in pancreatic β-cells resulting in the disappearance of 50% of these cells through apoptosis (Guo *et al.* 2007; Pick *et al.* 1998). This phenomenon of lipotoxicity can alter tissue function and cellular metabolism (DeFronzo 2010). Lipotoxicity associated with obesity and T2DM weakens β-cells via several causative agents, including ceramides, reactive oxygen species (ROS), inflammation and endoplasmic reticulum stress (Ye 2019).

Other mechanisms already mentioned before such as adipocytokines secreted by adipose tissue (TNFα, IL-6, adiponectin, etc.) may also explain this close link associating T2DM and obesity (Lee *et al.* 2019).

References

Aizawa, T., & Komatsu, M. (2005). Rab27a: a new face in β cell metabolism-secretion coupling. The Journal of clinical investigation, 115(2), 227-230.

Bergsten, P. (2000). Pathophysiology of impaired pulsatile insulin release. *Diabetes/Metabolism Research and Reviews*, *16*(3), 179-191.

Björnholm, M., & Zierath, J. R. (2005). Insulin signal transduction in human skeletal muscle: identifying the defects in Type II diabetes. Biochemical Society Transactions, 33(2), 354-357.

Buchanan, T. A. (2003). Pancreatic beta-cell loss and preservation in type 2 diabetes. *Clinical Therapeutics*, 25, B32-B46.

Campbell, J. E., & Newgard, C. B. (2021). Mechanisms controlling pancreatic islet cell function in insulin secretion. Nature Reviews Molecular Cell Biology, 22(2), 142-158.

Capeau, J. (2003). Insulin signalling pathways: mechanisms affected in insulin resistance. *Medicine/Science*, *19*(8-9), 834-839.

Chang, L., Chiang, S. H., & Saltiel, A. R. (2004). Insulin signaling and the regulation of glucose transport. Molecular medicine, 10(7), 65-71.

Coelho, M., Oliveira, T., Fernandes, R. (2013). Biochemistry of adipose tissue: An endocrine organ. Archive of Medicine Sciences, 9, 191-200.

DeFronzo, R. A., & Tripathy, D. (2009). Skeletal muscle insulin resistance is the primary defect in type 2 diabetes. *Diabetes care*, *32*(suppl_2), S157-S163.

DeFronzo, R. A. (2010). Insulin resistance, lipotoxicity, type 2 diabetes and atherosclerosis: the missing links. The Claude Bernard Lecture 2009. *Diabetologia*, *53*(7), 1270-1287.

Delarue, J., & Magnan, C. (2007). Free fatty acids and insulin resistance. *Current Opinion in Clinical Nutrition & Metabolic Care*, *10*(2), 142-148.

Flannery, C., Dufour, S., Rabøl, R., Shulman, G. I., & Petersen, K. F. (2012). Skeletal muscle insulin resistance promotes increased hepatic de novo lipogenesis, hyperlipidemia, and hepatic steatosis in the elderly. *Diabetes*, *61*(11), 2711-2717.

Gastaldelli, A., Baldi, S., Pettiti, M., Toschi, E., Camastra, S., Natali, A., ... Influence of obesity and type 2 diabetes on gluconeogenesis and glucose output in humans: a quantitative study. *Diabetes*, *49*(8), 1367-1373.

Griffin, M. E., Marcucci, M. J., Cline, G. W., Bell, K., Barucci, N., Lee, D., ... & Shulman, G. I. (1999). Free fatty acid-induced insulin resistance is associated with activation of protein kinase C theta and alterations in the insulin-signaling cascade. *Diabetes*, *48*(6), 1270-1274.

Guerre-Millo, M. (2004). Adipose tissue and adipokines: for better or worse. *Diabetes & metabolism*, *30*(1), 13-19.

Guillausseau, P. J., & Laloi-Michelin, M. (2003). Pathophysiology of type 2 diabetes. *La revue de médecine interne*, *24*(11), 730-737.

Jahandideh, F., & Wu, J. (2022). A review on mechanisms of action of bioactive peptides against glucose intolerance and insulin resistance. Food Science and Human Wellness, 11(6), 1441-1454.

Kahn, S. E., Prigeon, R. L., McCulloch, D. K., Boyko, E. J., Bergman, R. N., Schwartz, M. W., ... & Palmer, J. P. (1993). Quantification of the relationship between insulin sensitivity and β-cell function in human subjects: evidence for a hyperbolic function. *Diabetes*, *42*(11), 1663-1672.

Kim, J. H., Bachmann, R. A., & Chen, J. (2009). Interleukin-6 and insulin resistance. *Vitamins & Hormones*, *80*, 613-633.

Krogh-Madsen, R., Plomgaard, P., Møller, K., Mittendorfer, B., & Pedersen, B. K. (2006). Influence of TNF-α and IL-6 infusions on insulin sensitivity and expression of IL-18 in humans. *American Journal of Physiology-Endocrinology and Metabolism*, 291(1), E108-E114.

Leclercq, I. A., Morais, A. D. S., Schroyen, B., Van Hul, N., & Geerts, A. (2007). Insulin resistance in hepatocytes and sinusoidal liver cells: mechanisms and consequences. *Journal of hepatology*, 47(1), 142-156.

Lee, M. W., Lee, M., & Oh, K. J. (2019). Adipose tissue-derived signatures for obesity and type 2 diabetes: adipokines, batokines and microRNAs. *Journal of clinical medicine*, *8*(6), 854.

Marchetti, P., Dotta, F., Lauro, D., & Purrello, F. (2008). An overview of pancreatic beta-cell defects in human type 2 diabetes: implications for treatment. *Regulatory peptides*, 146(1-3), 4-11.

Muoio, D. M., & Newgard, C. B. (2008). Molecular and metabolic mechanisms of insulin resistance and β-cell failure in type 2 diabetes. *Nature reviews Molecular cell biology*, 9(3), 193-205.

Nguyen, T. V., Poole, D. P., Harvey, J. R., Stebbing, M. J., & Furness, J. B. (2005). Investigation of PKC isoform-specific translocation and targeting of the current of the late afterhyperpolarizing potential of myenteric AH neurons. *European Journal of Neuroscience*, 21(4), 905-913.

Permutt, M. A., Wasson, J., & Cox, N. (2005). Genetic epidemiology of diabetes. *The Journal of clinical investigation*, 115(6), 1431-1439.

Perry, R. J., Samuel, V. T., Petersen, K. F., & Shulman, G. I. (2014). The role of hepatic lipids in hepatic insulin resistance and type 2 diabetes. *Nature*, 510(7503), 84-91.

Petersen, K. F., & Shulman, G. I. (2006). Etiology of insulin resistance. *The American journal of medicine, 119*(5), S10-S16.

Petersen, M. C., & Shulman, G. I. (2018). Mechanisms of insulin action and insulin resistance. Physiological reviews, 98(4), 2133-2223.

Rabøl, R., Petersen, K. F., Dufour, S., Flannery, C., & Shulman, G. I. (2011). Reversal of muscle insulin resistance with exercise reduces postprandial hepatic de novo lipogenesis in insulin resistant individuals. *Proceedings of the National Academy of Sciences, 108*(33), 13705-13709.

Rosen, E. D., & Spiegelman, B. M. (2006). Adipocytes as regulators of energy balance and glucose homeostasis. *Nature, 444*(7121), 847-853.

Rutter, G. A., Pullen, T. J., Hodson, D. J., & Martinez-Sanchez, A. (2015). Pancreatic β-cell identity, glucose sensing and the control of insulin secretion. *Biochemical Journal*, 466(2), 203-218.

Samuel, V. T., Liu, Z. X., Qu, X., Elder, B. D., Bilz, S., Befroy, D., ... & Shulman, G. I. (2004). Mechanism of hepatic insulin resistance in non-alcoholic fatty liver disease. *Journal of Biological Chemistry, 279*(31), 32345-32353.

Steiner, D. F. (2000). New aspects of proinsulin physiology and pathophysiology. *Journal of pediatric endocrinology and metabolism, 13*(3), 229-240.

Temple, R., Clark, P. M. S., & Hales, C. N. (1992). Measurement of insulin secretion in type 2 diabetes: problems and pitfalls. *Diabetic medicine*, 9(6), 503-512.

Tokarz, V. L., MacDonald, P. E., & Klip, A. (2018). The cellular biology of systemic insulin function. *Journal of Cell Biology*, 217(7), 2273-2289.

Ye, R., Onodera, T., & Scherer, P. E. (2019). Lipotoxicity and β cell maintenance in obesity and type 2 diabetes. *Journal of the Endocrine Society*, 3(3), 617-631.

CHAPTER 3

TYPE 2 DIABETES: GENETIC ASPECT

T2DM is a multifactorial disease where genetic and environmental factors are closely associated. This form of diabetes presents extreme clinical and genetic heterogeneity, and its mode of transmission is in most cases unknown. The methods used to identify genes involved in T2DM are candidate gene approaches, genome-wide association studies (GWAS) and next generation sequencing (NGS) technology. These approaches have helped to identify more than 100 genetic variants linked to T2DM. However, these variants explain only part of the genetics of T2DM. Epigenetics, epistasis, gene-environment interactions, and non-coding RNAs are currently areas of research that provide a missing part of the genetic architecture of T2D.

1. Evidence for a genetic component in T2DM

1.1. Genetic epidemiology

The existence of genetic susceptibility factors for T2DM is suggested by different studies (Barroso 2005). Diabetes is characterised by a wide spectrum of prevalence in different ethnic groups. For example, among Mapuche Indians in Chile, T2DM is almost non-existent in the 30-64 age group, whereas among Pima Indians in Arizona, a prevalence of over 50% is observed in the same age group (King *et al.* 1993). In fact, in multi-ethnic populations, some ethnic groups not only have a much higher prevalence of diabetes than the same ethnic group living in the country of origin, but also a higher prevalence compared to other ethnic groups living in the same environment (Carulli *et al.* 2005). This suggests that some ethnic groups have a genetic predisposition to develop T2DM compared to others, when exposed to similar environmental conditions.

The presence of a type 2 diabetic in a family increases the risk of diabetes in other family members (Newman *et al.* 1987), which is in favour of a genetic involvement in the development of T2DM. Thus, a child has a 40% risk of developing T2DM if one parent has diabetes and 70% if both parents have diabetes (Groop & Tuomi 1997). In the Framingham Offspring Study, researchers found that if one parent has diabetes, the risk is increased in children by an odds ratio (OR) of 3.4-3.5, and if both parents are affected the risk is increased to 6.1 (Meigs *et al.* 2000). In addition, concordance studies between twins with at least one affected T2DM show a higher concordance in homozygotes (20%-91% depending on the study) than in heterozygotes (10%-43%) (Willemsen *et al.* 2015; Poulsen *et* al. 1999). This suggests strong genetic support for T2DM.

1.2. Monogenic forms of T2DM: MODYs

It is possible to differentiate families with T2DM according to the mode of transmission of the disease: polygenic diabetes, where the role of the environment is very important, and monogenic forms, where a mutation in a single gene is apparently sufficient to cause hyperglycaemia (Velho *et al.* 1997).

The monogenic forms appear very early in life, either at birth, in childhood or during adolescence. In general, these monogenic forms, which are called neonatal diabetes or MODY (Maturity Onset Type Diabetes of the Young), involve genes responsible for the primitive disorder of insulin secretion. Fourteen genetic mutations have been described so far affecting either the glucokinase gene for MODY 2 or the transcription factor genes HNF-1A, HNF-4A and HNF-1B for the MODY 3, 1, 5 forms, respectively (Table 2). The other forms are rarer (less than 1%) (Skoczek *et al.* 2021). They account for less than 5% of all T2DM cases (Urakami 2019).

Table 2. MODY diabetes genes. *According to* (Li *et al.* 2021)

Type	Gene	Pathophysiology
More common		
MODY3	HNF1A	β-cell dysfunction
MODY1	HNF4A	β-cell dysfunction
MODY5	HNF1B	β-cell dysfunction
MODY2	GCK	Genetic defect in glucokinase
Rare type		
MODY4	PDX1	β-cell dysfunction
MODY6	NEUROD1	β-cell dysfunction
MODY7	KLF11	β-cell dysfunction
MODY8	CEL	Exo-endocrine pancreatic insufficiency
MODY9	PAX4	β-cell dysfunction
MODY10	INS	Insulin gene mutation
MODY11	BLK	Insufficient insulin secretion
MODY12	ABCC8	ATP-dependent K channel dysfunction
MODY13	KCNJ11	ATP-dependent K channel dysfunction
MODY14	APPL1	Insufficient insulin secretion

1.3. Maternally transmitted T2DM: mitochondrial disease

A deletion of more than 10 kb of mitochondrial DNA has been described in a family with maternally inherited insulin-dependent diabetes associated with deafness (Ballinger *et al.* 1992). In a French study, a point mutation in mitochondrial DNA, co-segregating with T2DM and sensorineural hearing loss (called Maternally Inherited Diabetes and Deafness, MIDD), was found in 2% of families with T2DM (Vionnet *et al.* 1993). Other mutations have been found in the mitochondrial genome in families with diabetes (Maassen *et al.* 2005).

2. Evidence for an environmental component in T2DM

T2DM is caused by a combination of genetic and lifestyle factors. Although diabetes susceptibility genes are considered essential for the development of diabetes, their activation requires the presence of environmental factors, especially those related to lifestyle.

Various prospective epidemiological studies, including the well-known NHS Nurses' Health Study in the US, suggest that diet composition may play a role. A diet with a high glycaemic index, low in fibre and high in certain fatty acids (saturated and trans-unsaturated fats) doubles the risk of diabetes (Hu & Willett 2001). The overall analysis of the NHS results led to the conclusion that 90% of T2DM cases could be attributed to environmental factors (mainly overweight) and could therefore be prevented by a healthier lifestyle (Hu & Willett 2001). Recently, Schulze et al. found in the same cohort (NHS II) that women who consumed more than one sugar-sweetened soft drink per day had a relative risk (RR) of 1.83 for developing T2D (Schulze *et al.* 2004).

Other environmental factors such as the intrauterine environment can intervene very early in life and predispose to the onset of metabolic complications later in life. Indeed, it has been described that low birth weight but also high birth weight is associated with an increased risk for the development of T2DM in childhood (Whincup *et al.* 2008; Knop *et al.* 2018).

Disruption of sleep patterns and duration, and exposure to endocrine modulators have also been incriminated. Any average reduction of one hour of sleep would increase the risk of diabetes by 9%, exposure to tobacco by 30-60% and exposure to noise (10 dB) or fine particles (10 µg/m^3) by 20-40% (Kolb & Martin 2017).

3. Gene-environment interactions

The interaction between genes and environment in the genesis of T2DM is particularly well illustrated by the dramatic increase in the prevalence of the disease in certain well-defined ethnic groups following a change in their lifestyle. This is the case, for example, of the Pima Indians, who have one of the highest prevalence rates of obesity and T2D in the world (Knowler *et al.* 1990). These Arizona Indians experienced periods of famine at the beginning of the century which decimated a large part of their population. The survivors now live on reservations where they have access to a high-calorie Western diet. According to the 'sparing genotype' theory (Neel 1962), human history in general, and that of the Pima Indians in particular, has led to the natural selection of genes favourable to the survival of the species under the conditions of food deprivation that have prevailed for centuries. The individuals that survived would have metabolic characteristics that would allow them to store energy more efficiently and thus better resist starvation. Unfortunately, these same genes become a handicap in times of plenty, favouring diseases of plethora.

The increase in the prevalence of T2DM and obesity is due to changes in environmental habits and not to changes in genetic background. However, some environmental factors can only manifest their effects in the presence of certain genotypes (Fig. 10). Recently, epidemiological studies are trying to elucidate the molecular aspects of this interaction (Franks *et al.* 2007). For example, a variant of the PPAR-γ (Peroxisome-proliferated activator receptor gamma) gene appears to interact with the nature of high-fat dietary intake (Franks *et al.* 2007). Other interactions have been reported with adrenergic receptors, uncoupling proteins (UCP), apolipoproteins and lipoprotein lipase (Grarup & Andersen 2007; Franks *et al.* 2007).

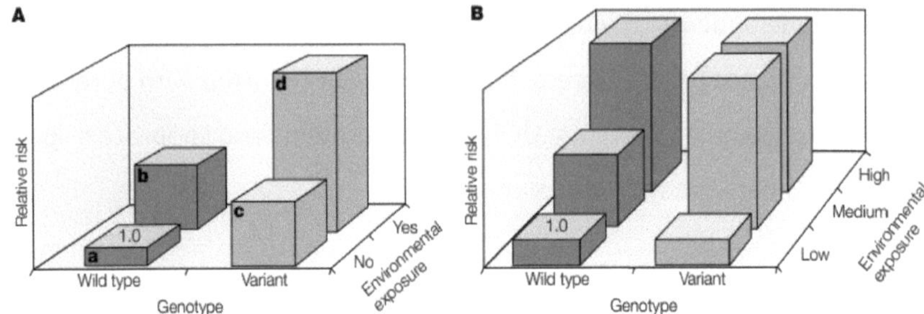

Figure 10: Model of gene-environment interactions. Adapted *from* (Hunter 2005).

These two figures illustrate the comparison of the relative risk of developing a disease between subjects carrying at least one risk allele and normal homozygous subjects, depending on whether or not they are exposed to permissive (disease) environmental factors. ***(A)*** *Column (a) is the reference column, and corresponds to a relative risk of 1. The relative risk of a disease is significantly higher in subjects carrying both the susceptibility allele and exposed to risky environmental factors (column d), compared to subjects carrying the risky allele and not exposed to the risky environment (c) or carrying the wild-type allele and exposed (b).* ***(B)*** *It has been proposed that genetically susceptible individuals are at risk despite low levels of exposure to permissive environmental factors. In this model, the difference in relative risk between genotypes in subjects with moderate exposure to permissive environmental factors for disease is evidence of gene-environment interactions.*

4. Genetic approaches to T2DM

The advent of modern molecular biology tools and their application to human genetics, as well as statistical methods, have led to a rapid and significant increase in knowledge, both about the aetiology of many hereditary diseases and about the functioning of living organisms, in the broadest sense (Mayeux 2005).

In contrast to monogenic forms, complex forms of T2DM can be defined as Mendelian defaulters, as they are instead determined by several susceptibility alleles distributed throughout the genome. These susceptibility factors have a reduced penetrance and only increase the risk of developing a disease that is otherwise largely dependent on the environment. Thus, susceptibility alleles for T2DM are often frequent in the general population and are also found in individuals without these diseases. The evaluation of the involvement of a polymorphism in the susceptibility to a complex disease is therefore done with the help of statistical analysis methods.

4.1. Molecular markers used in human genetics

DNA variations are stable and transmitted in a Mendelian fashion. They may be located in or near a gene and be in linkage disequilibrium with the pathogenic allele. These variations are therefore used as markers to identify mutations associated with or responsible for the diseased phenotype.

4.1.1. RFLP markers

The first generation of genetic markers is represented in particular by RFLPs (Restriction Fragment Length Polymorphisms). The principle of RFLPs is based on the unique property of highly specific recognition of bacterial restriction site endonucleases which, depending on the presence or absence of a polymorphism, generate fragments of variable size. These markers enabled one of the first genetic linkage studies in humans (Botstein *et al.* 1980). Later, genetic markers generated by PCR (Polymerase Chain Reaction) also represented a huge advance in the field of genetic studies. The PCR technique consists of denaturing the DNA into a single-stranded form, attaching primers and polymerising it with Taq DNA polymerase. The three temperatures and their application times are managed by a thermal cycler. Theoretically, any genomic sequence could be studied from very small amounts of DNA and, therefore, at a lower cost than with RFLP markers (Avise 2012).

Two types of markers have proven to be particularly useful in human genetics: microsatellite markers and SNPs.

4.1.2. Microsatellite markers

On the genome, there are DNA sequences characterised by (CA)n (cytosine-adenosine) tandem dinucleotide repeats (where $12<n<75$) approximately every 25 to 100 kilobases, these are the microsatellites (Ellegren 2004). Characterised by a specific flanking sequence, their amplification by PCR makes it possible to determine the number of repeats they contain and thus defines the allele.

This number of repeats is variable in DNA populations and within an individual's alleles. The sequence below has a 20 dinucleotide (40 bp) repeat sequence of CA which is shown in bold.

CGTTCAATAAGCAAAAATCCATAGTTAGGAATGTGGGCT GCTTGGTGTGATGTAGAAGGCGCCAATGCATCTCGACGTAT **GCGTATACGGGTTACCCCCTTTGCAATCAGTGCACACACA** CACACACACACACACACACACACACACAGTGCCAAGCAA AAATAACGCCAAGCAGAACGAAGACGTTCTCGAGAACACCA GAAGTTCGTGCTGTCGGGGCATGCGGCGAGTAAAGGGGAT

When a microsatellite is flanked by fluorescent PCR primers, the amplification will result in a pair of fluorescent allelic products whose size will vary according to their repeat length.

These markers are highly polymorphic and have quickly become a widely used tool in genetic linkage studies within families and linkage disequilibrium studies of populations (Al-Samarai & Al-Kazaz 2015).

Studies have shown that a group of candidate microsatellites could be detected by intergenomic comparisons against a specific functional gene cluster, and successful identification would reveal polymorphic microsatellites in functional domains and thus facilitate experimental designs for various biological applications (Pai & Chen 2016).

4.1.3. Bi-allelic markers or Single Nucleotid Polymophism (SNP)

SNPs are the most common bi-allelic sequence polymorphisms and are observed on average once every 1000 bp in the genome. Currently, 81 million SNPs have been identified in the human genome (The 1000 Genomes Project Consortium 2015). Most of these SNPs are rare alleles with frequencies of less than 1% (68.4 million SNPs in 1000 genomes).

A SNP is considered to be frequent if the rare allele is present in at least 5% of the healthy subjects studied. When SNPs are present in the regulatory sites of a gene, they cause changes in the production of the encoded protein. In the coding regions, SNPs can cause alterations in the structure of proteins and thus lead to the development of a disease. Thus, SNPs have been used as molecular markers in many genetic diseases (Kim & Misra 2007). The major advantage of SNPs is that they can be genotyped in a very large number of individuals at a relatively low cost. The most reliable method for identifying a SNP is direct sequencing. This is also true for genotyping (Chang *et al.* 2009). Within the genome, SNPs are grouped into several linkage disequilibrium (LD) blocks. Linkage disequilibrium corresponds to the non-random joint segregation on a chromosome of two or more alleles from two or more different loci at a higher frequency than would be expected by chance, i.e. the information gathered on one SNP is valid for all SNPs in the block (depending on the strength of the LD). This will allow one SNP per LD block to be genotyped without losing genetic information, in order to reduce the cost of genotyping.

4.2. Association studies

4.2.1. Case-control study

In diseases with complex inheritance, association studies for a gene consist of assessing the correlation between polymorphisms in that gene and the disease using appropriate statistical tools (Rao 2001). Case-control studies are retrospective studies that look for a difference in allele or genotype frequency between a group of subjects with the disease of interest and a group of subjects without the disease. The subjects should all be unrelated and of the same ethnic origin. Ideally, the two groups should be matched for sex and age.

In a case-control study, the effect of a SNP is measured by the odds ratio (OR), which compares the frequency of the risk allele in the two groups of subjects (Table 3). The χ test² (chi-2) estimates whether the frequency of the tested variant is significantly different between the affected and unaffected group at the α risk of 5%. If the mutated or "rare" allele is more frequent in affected subjects, it is called a "risk allele". On the contrary, if this mutated allele is more frequent in control subjects, it is called a "protective" allele.

Table 3: Calculation of the OR in case-control analysis

	Carrier of the A allele	Carrier of the B allele
Cases	a	b
Witnesses	c	d

OR = a×d / c×b where: a = frequency of the A allele in the cases
b = frequency of the B allele in the cases
c = frequency of the A allele in controls
d = frequency of the B allele in controls

There are many methodological biases in association studies that are thought to be responsible for the lack of replication of results (Healy 2006; Cordell & Clayton 2005).

The first bias is related to the phenotype. Thus, choosing a homogeneous group of patients requires a standard definition of the diagnostic criteria and the etiology of the disease.

The second bias is related to lack of statistical power (Redden & Allison 2003). Indeed, the lack of replication of associations in several studies may reflect a lack of statistical power that wrongly concludes that no associations actually exist. Thus, accurate assessment of the often modest effects of complex disease susceptibility variants requires the use of large numbers of subjects (Wang *et al.* 2005) (Fig. 11).

A third bias is related to population stratification, which is the most cited cause of the lack of replication of genetic association results. The existence of stratification in a population corresponds to variations in allele frequency and disease prevalence among subgroups that make up the study population (Redden & Allison 2003). Thus, if such differences are not known to exist, an association between a genetic polymorphism and a disease in that population would reflect differences between these subgroups of individuals rather than a true cause of predisposition (Cardon & Palmer 2003).

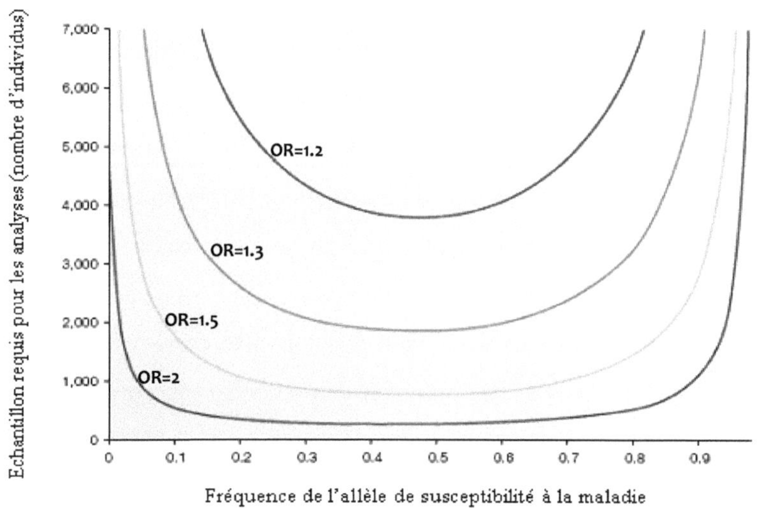

Figure 11: Size of the population to be genotyped in association studies (based on SNP frequency and strength of association). Adapted from (Wang *et al.* 2005).

The number of case and control subjects required to identify a disease susceptibility variant with an allelic OR of 1.2 to 2 is shown on the y-axis. The number of subjects required is shown to achieve a statistical power of 80% and a significance level <10⁻ . [6]For example, if the risk variant has an allelic frequency of less than 0.1 and its OR is 1.3, a population of more than 10,000 cases and 10,000 controls is required to detect the association.

As association analysis is very sensitive to genotyping errors and stratification bias, it is important after each genotyping to check the Hardy Weinberg equilibrium. For 2 alleles A and B of frequencies p and 1-p respectively, this test assumes that the alleles are randomly distributed to form the genotypes, with the following distribution (homozygous wild type, heterozygous and homozygous mutated): $p + 2pq + q^{22} = 1$. A deviation from the Hardy-Weinberg equilibrium may be due to genotyping error, mixing of subpopulations (or *stratification bias*) within the study population or selection phenomena. Under particular genetic models, an imbalance in affected individuals may indicate a marker effect, and thus an association. Finally, it should not be forgotten that a deviation from equilibrium may be due to chance, depending on the number of SNPs tested.

In addition, several methods have been developed to correct for bias and validate association results. The Bonferroni correction consists of dividing the classical threshold of 0.05 by the number of tests performed (or *the number of null hypotheses*) in the same sample (Colhoun *et al.* 2003). However, these purely statistical methods are very conservative and are likely to generate an even higher number of false negative results (Redden & Allison 2003). Thus, taking into consideration the biological meaning of the association and, most importantly, independently replicating the association in the original publication are accepted ways to validate a genetic association result (Little *et al.* 2009). It is not excluded that an association is not replicated in a population simply because the SNP studied is in LD with the true causative polymorphism. Thus, because of the difference in LOD between populations, a significant association may or may not be observed (Colhoun *et al.* 2003; Redden & Allison 2003; Little *et al.* 2009).

Meta-analyses are mainly used to pool observations and thus improve the precision in estimating the association of a variant. These meta-analyses help to avoid bias due to lack of statistical power. Stratification is undoubtedly the weak point of case-control studies (Redden & Allison 2003). Therefore, family association studies can complement and validate a result obtained from case-control analysis.

4.2.2. Transmission imbalance tests (TDT)

The TDT (Transmission Disequilibrium Test) was developed by Spielman and colleagues for the analysis of qualitative traits, such as association analysis in families with at least one affected descendant as well as both parents (Spielman *et al.* 1993). The principle of this test is based on the detection of an excess or a defect in the transmission of the rare allele from a heterozygous parent to an affected child compared to the theoretical 50% rate (Fig. 12) (Spielman *et al.* 1993). The existence of such a bias is interpreted as an association between the allele of interest and the disease. Analysis of the transmission of the allele in question in a general population would make it possible to distinguish between a distortion intrinsic to this polymorphism and a distortion associated with the disease (Eaves *et al.* 1999). Apart from the great advantage of excluding stratification bias, the advantage of this test is that it tests for both linkage and association (Laird & Lange 2006) and is applicable in both quantitative and binary trait analysis (Zhang *et al.* 2003).

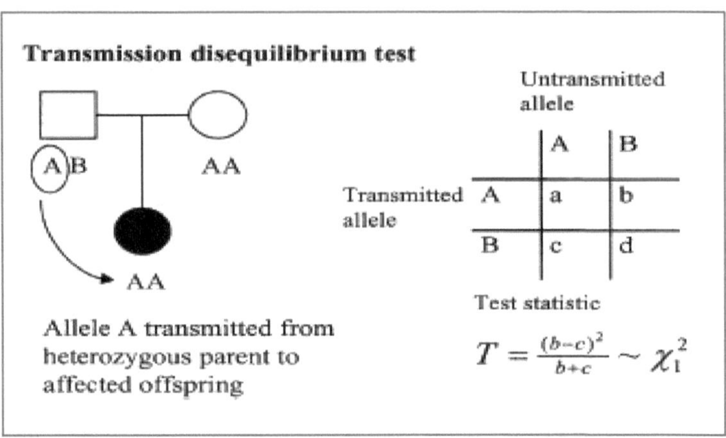

Figure 12: TDT diagram and statistical test.

The TDT test is based on trio families (both parents and the affected child) with known genotypes. In many trios, this test compares the observed number of A alleles transmitted to the affected child with those expected in normal Mendelian transmission. An excess of the A (or B) allele among affected children indicates that the marker tested is linked and in linkage disequilibrium with the locus of susceptibility to the disease or trait tested. In the figure, the mother can only transmit the A allele knowing that she is homozygous for the A allele, however, the father being heterozygous, can transmit the A and B allele at equal frequencies resulting in AA or AB children at equal frequencies. The TDT test eliminates all homozygous parents and tests only for transmission from the heterozygous parent to the affected child. The T-test compares the number of transmissions of the A and B alleles and follows a χ distribution² with one degree of freedom.

The problem with this test is that in late-onset diseases such as T2DM, it is sometimes difficult to access the genotypes of the parents of affected individuals. In addition, a relatively low frequency of a variant may result in low statistical power as only heterozygous parents in the trios analysed are informative. An alternative method in which parental genotypes are replaced by the genotypes of unaffected siblings is the Sibship Disequilibrium Test (SDT) method (Horvath & Laird 1998). The number of deleterious alleles carried by the affected members is compared to the number of deleterious alleles carried by the unaffected. The resulting statistic follows a χ distribution^{2} .

4.3. Haplotype studies

The study of individual effects of polymorphisms on susceptibility to a multifactorial disease can be complemented by haplotype analysis. The haplotype is defined by the combination of several alleles belonging to different loci transmitted together within the same chromosome (Crawford and Nickerson 2005). These studies can also detect the effect of a functional mutation that is not genotyped and is in strong linkage disequilibrium with the haplotype. It is also possible to test the familial association (TDT) of haplotypes and study their effects on quantitative and qualitative traits. Furthermore, multi-SNP haplotypes provide a more accurate view of the genomic structure of the polymorphic population than individual SNPs (Vadva *et al.* 2019).

4.4. Analysis of phenotypes associated with T2D

The concept 'phenotype' is beginning to attract the attention of philosophers of biology as the case of 'genotype' (Nachtomy *et al.* 2007). The correct definition of the phenotype is an important condition for the performance of a genetic study. T2DM is a complex and heterogeneous disease. Analysis of intermediate phenotypes, more precise than the diabetic versus non-diabetic dichotomy based on blood glucose thresholds, such as insulin resistance, pancreatic β-cell performance and mass, BMI index and other features of the metabolic syndrome would increase our chances of identifying susceptibility genes (Meigs 2019; Permutt *et al.* 2005).

The effect of genetic variants on these quantitative traits is tested using tests of comparisons of means. For some intermediate phenotypes, it is difficult to distinguish between a causative and a consequential effect of the phenotypic variation on the disease. It is recommended to study the effect of the variants on phenotypes close to the physiological function of the genes harbouring them, thus reducing the effect due to disease heterogeneity (Lander & Schork 2006). For example, a variant in the resistin promoter has been shown to be associated with T2DM and elevated fasting resistin levels (Osawa *et al.* 2004) and SNPs in the adiponectin promoter have been shown to predispose to hypoadiponectinemia and T2DM (Vasseur *et al.* 2005).

4.5. Gene-gene interaction or epistasis studies

Due to the lack of statistical power, which is a major obstacle, gene-gene interaction studies are not widely addressed in genetic studies. However, their role is crucial in the determination of complex diseases. About ten studies on one or more phenotypes have attempted to elucidate the combined effect of two or more polymorphisms. For example, Qi et al.

studied the effect of epistasis on T2DM in women participating in the NHS study (Qi *et al.* 2007). In this study, two predisposing variants for T2DM were investigated, the P2 variant of the transcription factor hepatocyte nuclear factor 4 alpha (*HNF4A*) gene promoter and the E23K variant of the B-cell ATP-sensitive K^+ channel subunit Kir6.2 (*KCNJ11*) gene. According to the results of this study, there is a significant interaction between 3 SNPs of the *HNF4A* gene and the E23K of the *KCNJ11* gene. In another study, Weedon et al. did not find a significant gene-gene interaction between the Lys23 variant of the *KCNJ11* gene, the Pro12 variant of the *PPARG* (peroxisome proliferator-activated receptors gamma) gene and the T allele in rs7903146 of the *TCF7L2* (transcription factor 7-like 2) gene, despite their strong associations with T2DM (Weedon *et al.* 2006). In another large study, Cauchi et al. demonstrated that genes expressed in the pancreas interact with each other and their combined effect significantly increases the risk of T2DM (Cauchi *et al.* 2008).

4.6. Candidate gene approach

The candidate gene approach is widely used for the identification of polymorphisms involved in susceptibility to complex genetic diseases. The methodology of this approach is simple: first designate a gene and identify one (or more) genetic marker(s), then obtain for this (these) marker(s) genotypes in large populations. Finally, test whether there is a correlation between the genotype studied and the disease or disease-related phenotypes using case-control and/or family association analysis.

The critical step is the choice of the candidate gene. This choice may be based on the state of scientific knowledge regarding the pathophysiology of the disease, and is referred to as a "physiological candidate gene". Physiological arguments can be derived from the results of *in vivo* or *in vitro* studies. When the tissue-specific global invalidation of a gene, or its overexpression in the animal model, results in obesity, insulin resistance and/or diabetes, these are strong arguments for studying the role played by the gene in question in the susceptibility to these pathologies in humans (Ktorza *et al.* 1997). Other types of studies, such as antibody neutralisation, expression blocking with antisense oligonucleotides or RNA interference, interaction studies in signalling pathways or tissue-specific expression analyses, are prime sources for the identification of candidate genes for T2DM susceptibility.

A new approach has been developed based on the candidate gene approach and is called DigiCGA (digital candidate gene approach) (Zhu & Zhao 2007). It is an approach that is based on the extraction, filtration, clustering and analysis of all available public data resources on the web in accordance with the principles of biological ontology and statistical methods to identify potential candidate genes.

4.7. Genome-wide study

A whole genome study requires the genotyping of markers evenly distributed across the genome in a large number of families or populations. Then, the link between the markers and the disease is calculated using statistical tools adapted to the study of complex diseases. This is possible thanks to the existence of physical maps of the human genome. In this respect, microsatellite markers have been widely used because of their high genetic informativeness (existence of a large number of alleles for the same locus). However, SNPs are gradually replacing microsatellite markers as a molecular tool in whole genome studies. Indeed, SNPs have the advantage of providing denser and more accurate physical maps, which allows for better extraction of genetic information (Evans & Cardon 2004).

Two types of family samples can be used to conduct a whole genome study. Families from the general population, especially in ethnic groups with a very high prevalence of obesity, are a powerful way to study genetic linkage to quantitative traits associated with obesity, insulin resistance and T2DM (Bell *et al.* 2005). The second type of family chosen for this type of study corresponds to families with a recurrence of the disease (Bell *et al.* 2005). In this case, genetic linkage between a marker and the disease is suggested if the affected sib-pairs share significantly more IBD (identical by descent) alleles than expected by chance (Blackwelder *et al.* 1985).

The genome-wide study based on association studies has several advantages for identifying gene variants associated with common diseases (Hirschhorn & Daly 2005). This approach represents a comprehensive, unbiased method even in the absence of well-determined causal gene function or location.

The first genome-wide association study (GWAS) for T2DM (Sladek *et al.* 2007) demonstrated the importance of this type of approach in complex diseases. With a relatively small sample size (694 cases and 645 controls), their design allowed them to identify the *TCF7L2* gene variant, as well as a non-synonymous SNP in the zinc transporter *SLC30A8* and variants in the *HHEX* gene. This study was immediately followed by a series of genome-wide analyses, including the deCODE Genetics study (Steinthorsdottir *et al.* 2007), the Wellcome Trust Case Control Consortium (WTCCC) study (Zeggini *et al.* 2007), the Diabetes Genetics Initiative (DGI) study (Saxena *et al.* 2007) and the FUSION study (Scott *et al.* 2007). Subsequently, until 2010, different studies around the world defined 44 variants associated with T2DM (Fig. 13).

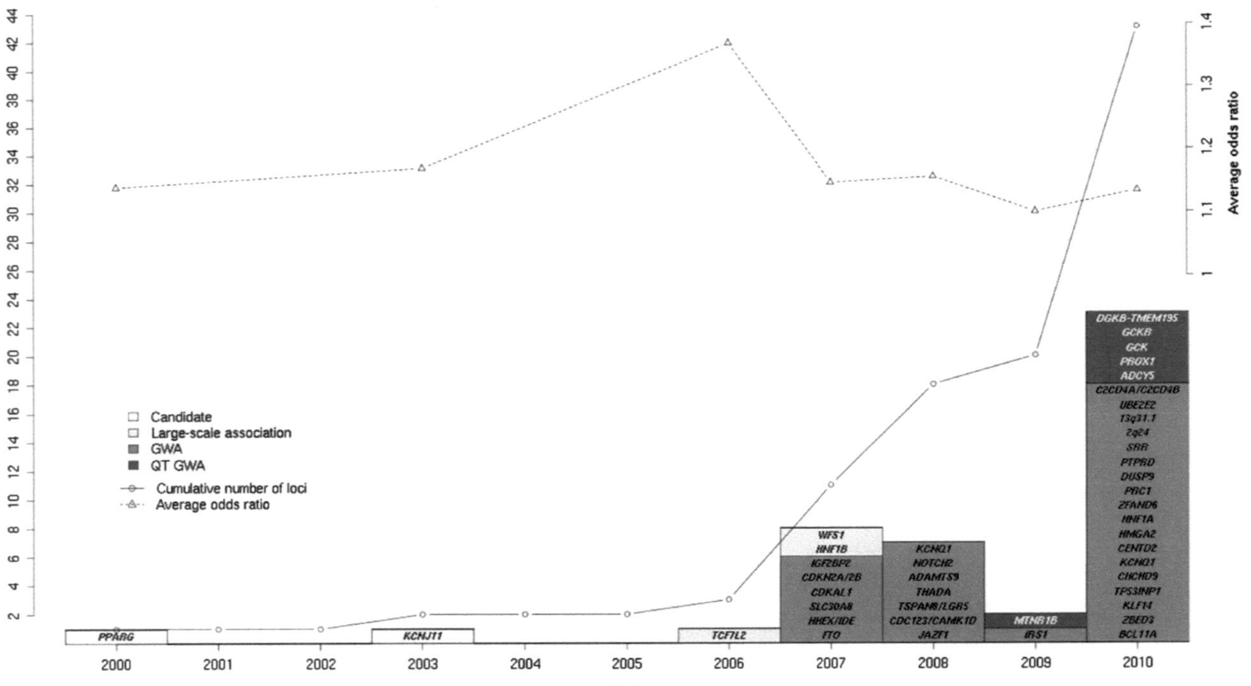

Figure 13: Identification of variants associated with T2D: A timeline of methods (Wheeler & Barroso 2011).

Polygenic risk scores (PRS) propose to express in a single numerical value the capacity of a given genome to produce a complex trait. These scores become analytical and predictive tools that are supposed to reflect the genetic potential of an individual with respect to these traits, calculated on the basis of the genotypic profile and relevant data from GWAS studies (Dheur & Saupe 2020; Choi *et al.* 2020).

Taking advantage of data from existing large-scale genome-wide association studies, polygenic risk scores have shown promise in complementing the list of clinical risk factors and intervention paradigms established to improve early diagnosis and prevention of T2DM (Ge *et al.* 2022). Thus, great efforts are being made to integrate PRS T2DM data into primary health care (Mars *et al.* 2022; Ge *et al.* 2022: Guinan *et al.* 2021).

Recently, a genome-wide multi-ethnic study identified 237 loci with a highly significant association with T2DM ($p < 5 \times 10^{-9}$), which were delineated into 338 distinct association signals (Mahajan *et al.* 2022) (Fig. 14). This study compiles statistical data from 122 GWAS studies with 180,834 T2DM cases and 1,159,055 controls in five ethnic groups: European, East Asian, South Asian, Hispanic and African.

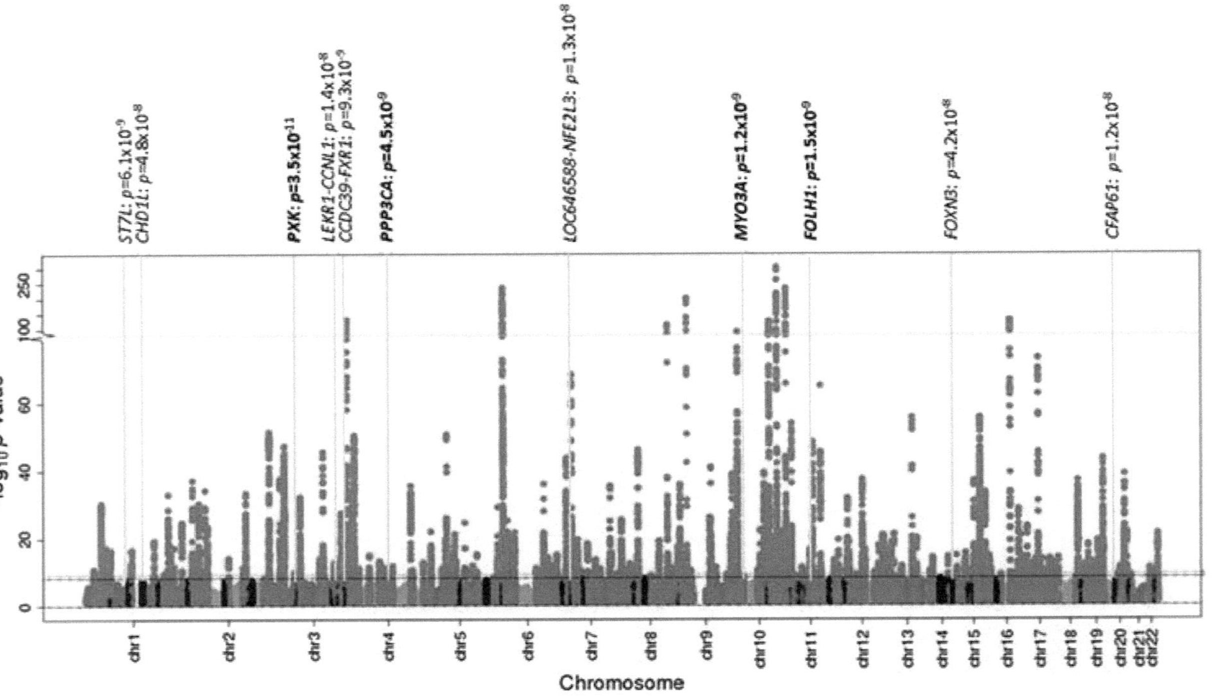

Figure 14: Manhattan plot of T2DM variants from multi-ethnic meta-regression. Adapted from (Mahajan *et al.* 2022). *New loci are highlighted with their significance value.*

5. Genes associated with T2D

The identification, through genetic analysis, of genes involved in disease development represents a powerful strategy for revealing the key pathways and mechanisms responsible for predisposition and progression. Indeed, a good definition of the etiology of T2DM will lead to new therapeutic avenues and more individualised interventions and treatments. On the other hand, genetics is an important approach in predicting diseases with complex inheritance. Thus, the usefulness of intervention in a population at risk of developing T2DM, by genetic information, has been illustrated in a prospective study in glucose intolerant people (Florez *et al.* 2006).

Advances in the genomics of T2DM are the result of the availability of data from GWAS studies. The development of genotyping platforms, the compilation of SNP databases, the building of large patient cohorts and the development of new sophisticated analytical methods contribute directly to the success of such studies. These studies produce between 70% and 80% of the variation in the human genome (Moore & Florez 2008).

In 2007, in addition to the three known genes associated with T2DM, six new genes were identified by five new GWAS studies (Sladek *et al.* 2007; Saxena *et al.* 2007; Steinthorsdottir *et al.* 2007; Scott *et al.* 2007; Zeggini *et al.* 2007) (Tables 4A and 4B). The number of variants associated with T2DM has increased over time. The large amount of data from GWAS studies has identified more than 250 variants associated with T2DM (Dornbos *et al.* 2020). Recently, in a multi-ethnic meta-analysis, with 228,499 cases and 1,178,783 controls, encompassing 5 ethnic groups (European, African American, Hispanic, South Asian and East Asian), researchers identified 804 putative causal genes at newly and previously reported loci (Vujkovic *et al.* 2020). Of these, 54 genes were found to be possible targets for drugs approved by the US Food and Drug Administration.

Table 4A: Characteristics of the 5 GWAS studies in type 2 diabetes and their replications

Studies (2007)	Case (n)	Controls (n)	Population	Confirmed genes
Sladek *et al.*	661	614	France	
Replication	2617	2894	France	*TCF7L2, SLC30A8, HHEX*
Saxena *et al.*	1464	1467	Finland, Sweden	
Replication	5065	5785	Sweden, Poland, USA	*TCF7L2, CDKAL1, CDKN2A/B, HHEX, SLC30A8, IGF2BP2, FTO, PPARG, KCNJ11*
Steinthorsdottir *et al.*	1399	5275	Iceland	
Replication	3826	12562	Denmark, Philadelphia, Holland	*TCF7L2, CDKAL1, SLC30A8, HHEX*
Scott *et al.*	1161	1174	Finland	
Replication	1215	1258	Finland	*TCF7L2, CDKAL1, CDKN2A/B, HHEX, SLC30A8, IGF2BP2, FTO, PPARG, KCNJ11*
Zeggini *et al.*	1924	2938	UK	
Replication	3757	5346	UK	*TCF7L2, CDKAL1, CDKN2A/B, HHEX, SLC30A8, IGF2BP2, FTO, PPARG, KCNJ11*

TCF7L2: Transcription Factor 7-like 2; *CDKAL1*: CDK5 regulatory subunit associated protein L-like 1; *CDKN2A/B*: Cyclin-Dependent kinase inhibitor 2A/B; *HHEX*: Hematopoietically Expressed Homeobox; *SLC30A8*: Solute Carrier family 30 (zinc transporter) member 8; *IGF2BP2*: Insulin-like Growth Factor 2 mRNA Binding Protein 2; *FTO*: Fat mass and Obesity; *PPARG*: Peroxisome Proliferator-Activated Receptor Gamma; *KCNJ11*: potassium inwardly-rectifying channel subfamily J member 11

Table 4B: Genes identified by the 5 GWAS studies in T2DM and their characteristics

			Sladek *et al* (n = 6794)	**Steinthorsdottir *et al* (*n* = 10056)**	**DGI (*n* =13781)**	**WTCCC (*n* = 13965)**	**Scott *et al.* (*n* = 4808)**	**Meta-analysis (*n* = 32554)**
SNP	**Gene**	**Chr**	OR (*p*)	OR (*p*)	OR (*p*)	OR (*p*)	OR (*p*)	OR (*p*)
rs7903146	*TCF7L2*	10	1.65 (3.3.10)$^{-10}$	1.38 (1.9.10)$^{-10}$	1.38 (2.3.10)$^{-31}$	1.37 (6.7.10)$^{-13}$	1.34 (1.4.10)$^{-8}$	1.37 (1.0.10)$^{-48}$
rs5219	*KCNJ11*	11	1,34 (0,074)	-	1.15 (1.0.10)$^{-7}$	1.15 (1.3.10)$^{-3}$	1,11 (0,014)	1.14 (6.7.10)$^{-11}$
rs1801282	*PPARG*	3	1,22 (0,11)	-	1,09 (0,019)	1.23 (1.3.10)$^{-3}$	1.20 (1.4.10)$^{-3}$	1.14 (1.7.10)$^{-6}$
rs4402960	*IGF2BP2*	3	-	-	1.17 (1.7.10)$^{-9}$	1.11 (1.6.10)$^{-4}$	1.18 (2.4.10)$^{-4}$	1.14 (8.9.10)$^{-16}$
rs10811661	*CDKN2B*	9	-	-	1.20 (5.4.10)$^{-8}$	1.19 (4.9.10)$^{-7}$	1.20 (2.2.10)$^{-3}$	1.20 (7.8.10)$^{-15}$
rs7754840	*CDKAL1*	6	-	1.2 (7.7.10)$^{-9}$	1.08 (2.4.10)$^{-3}$	1.16 (1.3.10)$^{-8}$	1.12 (9.5.10)$^{-3}$	1.12 (4.1.10)$^{-11}$
rs1111875	*HHEX*	10	1.21 (8.6.10)$^{-6}$	1,17 (0,001)	1.14 (1.7.10)$^{-4}$	1.13 (4.6.10)$^{-6}$	1,10 (0,025)	1.13 (5.7.10)$^{-10}$
rs13266634	*SLC30A8*	8	1.18 (5.0×10)$^{-7}$	1,19 (0,001)	1,07 (0,047)	1.12 (7.0.10)$^{-5}$	1.18 (7.0.10)$^{-5}$	1.12 (5.3.10)$^{-8}$

* Meta-analysis of studies: DGI, WTCCC and Scott *et al*; Chr: chromosome; OR: odds ratio

5.1. Transcription factor 7-like 2 (*TCF7L2*)

In early 2006, Grant et al. published an association between T2DM and a transcription factor 7-like 2 (*TCF7L2)* intron 3 microsatellite in a case-control sample from Iceland (Grant *et al.* 2006). Linkage disequilibrium was found between the variant and two single-nucleotide polymorphisms (SNPs) rs12255372 and rs7903146, with a close and similar association of these with T2DM ($p<10^{-15}$). Compared to non-carriers, heterozygous and homozygous carriers of the risk-conferring alleles (38% and 7% of the Icelandic population, respectively) had a relative risk of diabetes of 1.45 and 2.41. This corresponds to a population attributable risk of 21%. This association is not unique to Icelanders. Studies in European and American Caucasians, East Indians, Afro-Caribbeans, Chinese, Moroccans, Japanese and Emiratis of both sexes have confirmed the 'global' distribution of the *TCF7L2-DT2* association (Florez *et al.* 2006; Zhang *et al.* 2006; Scott *et al.* 2006; Cauchi *et al.* 2006; Bodhini *et al.* 2007; Cauchi *et al.* 2007; Miyake *et al.* 2008; Saadi *et al.* 2008). It has been suggested that polymorphisms in the *TCF7L2* gene are involved in up to one-fifth of cases of type 2 diabetes (Tong *et al.* 2009).

Over the years, several polymorphisms of the *TCF7L2* gene have been identified in studies of different diseases (del Bosque-Plata *et al.* 2022). The most common variants of the *TCF7L2* gene have been associated with various human diseases (Table 5).

Table 5: Most common *TCF7L2* gene variants with pleiotropic effects in human diseases (del Bosque-Plata *et al.* 2022)

TCF7L2-SNP	Diseases
rs7903146	T2D; T1D; GDM; LADA; increases risk of T2D by affecting glycaemic index in obese and non-obese subjects;

TCF7L2-SNP	Diseases
	increases risk of hypertension in T2D diabetics; diabetic nephropathy; cancer; schizophrenia; *cystic fibrosis*; precocious puberty; PCOS; cardiovascular disease
rs12255372	T2D; LADA; increases risk of T2D by affecting glycaemic index in overweight and non-overweight subjects; increases glycaemic index and risk of T2D in patients with metabolic syndrome; cancer; cardiovascular disease
rs7901695	T2DM; diabetic nephropathy

GDM, gestational diabetes; LADA, latent autoimmune diabetes in adults; PCOS, polycystic ovary syndrome

The human *TCF7L2* gene is located on chromosome 10q25.3 and was originally sequenced in colorectal cancer cell lines (Duval *et al.* 2000). The *TCF7L2* gene consists of 18 exons and contains highly conserved sequences that correspond to functional domains (Fig. 15). The β-catenin binding domain corresponds to exon 1 and the HMG box binding domain corresponds to exons 10 and 11 of human *TCF7L2* (del Bosque-Plata *et al.* 2021). Both domains are highly conserved between species.

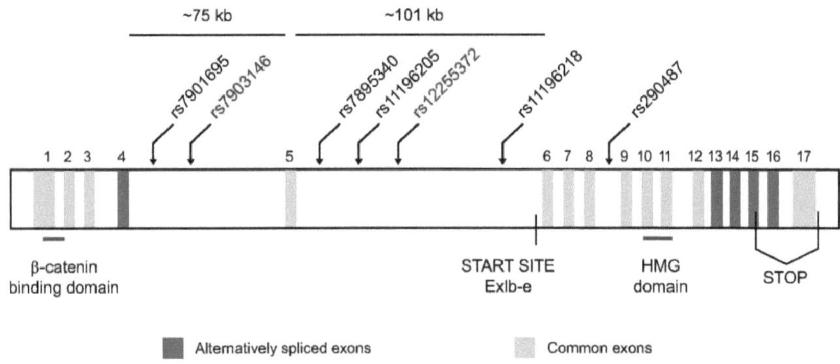

Figure 15: Structure of the *TCF7L2* gene. *Adapted* from (del Bosque-Plata *et al.* 2021)

Grant et al. proposed that *TCF7L2* variants increase the risk of developing T2DM by being likely to act via the regulation of proglucagon gene expression in endocrine cells of the gastrointestinal tract through the Wnt signalling pathway (Grant *et al.* 2006; Grant 2019). Furthermore, several studies have demonstrated the involvement of the Wnt signalling pathway in the development of the endocrine pancreas and the modulation of mature β-cell functions including insulin secretion, survival and proliferation (del Bosque-Plata *et al.* 2021; Chen *et al.* 2021) (Fig. 16).

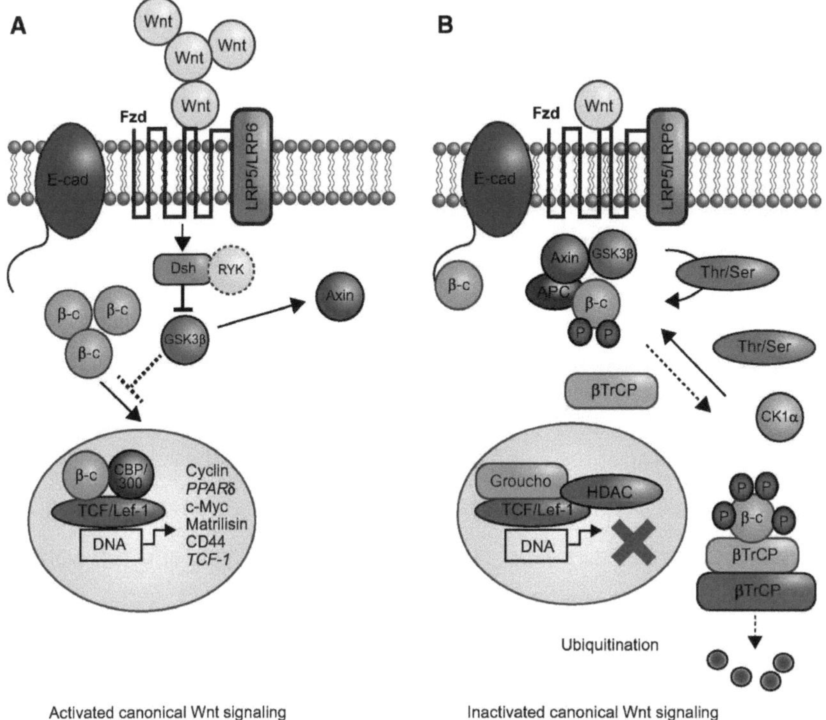

Figure 16: Wnt signal transmission pathway. Adapted from (del Bosque-Plata *et al.* 2021).

*(**A**) β-catenin protein is degraded in cells not exposed to Wnt protein. (**B**) When Wnt proteins bind to the Frizzeled receptor, β-catenin accumulates in the cytoplasm and then migrates to the nucleus where it can heterodimerise with TCF/LEF family transcription factors and activate the target gene.*

APC: adenomatous polyposis coli; GSK3: glycogen synthase kinase 3; LRP: low-density lipoprotein receptor-related protein; Dsh: disheveled; Lef: lymphoid enhancer factor; Tcf: T-cell factor

Another possible role for *TCF7L2* is its involvement in insulin secretion. Thus, after their studies on isolated human islets, Lyssenko et al. proposed that the risk allele increases *TCF7L2* expression in pancreatic β-cells, decreases insulin secretion and thereby leads to T2DM (Lyssenko *et al.* 2007). Shu et al. also reported that changes in circulating or active *TCF7L2* levels in pancreatic β-cells may contribute to impaired insulin secretion and the development of T2D (Shu *et al.* 2009).

In a study by Le Bacquer *et al* (2011), through an analysis of isolated human islets, three explanations were provided for the impact of the *TCF7L2* gene on β-cell function and survival. While *TCF7L2* clone B1, lacking exons 13, 14, 15 and 16, induces β-cell apoptosis, impairs function and inhibits the response of GLP-1 receptor agonists and downstream targets of Wnt signalling, clones B3 and B7, which both contain exon 13, enhance β-cell function and survival and activate the Wnt signalling pathway. (ii) *TCF7L2* gene mRNA is highly unstable and rapidly degraded under pro-diabetic conditions and (iii) *TCF7L2* depletion in islets induces *GSK3-β* (glycogen synthase kinase 3-β) gene activation, but this was independent of endoplasmic reticulum stress.

5.2. Peroxisome proliferator activated receptorγ (PPAR)γ

PPARγ has been the target of numerous association studies for susceptibility to the metabolic syndrome, given its major role in the maintenance of lipid and carbohydrate homeostasis. In 1998, Deeb and colleagues were the first to describe a specific mutation in the *PPARγ2* isoform (Deeb *et al.* 1998). This mutation consists of a change from Proline to Alanine associated with protection against T2DM, improved insulin sensitivity and reduced BMI. Since then, many studies have attempted to replicate these original associations, but the results were controversial (Gouda *et al.* 2010). In the Arab population, this variant is not associated with T2D (Meyer *et al.* 2009; O'Beirne *et al.* 2016).

In 2000, Altshuler et al. conducted a meta-analysis of 16 positive associations with T2DM, BMI, insulin levels and fasting blood glucose, and confirmed the role of Pro12Ala in T2DM susceptibility (Altshuler *et al.* 2000). A prospective French study, which was conducted in 3,914 individuals of Caucasian origin, tested, among other things, the association of the Pro12Ala variant with parameters related to insulin resistance and the incidence of impaired glucose tolerance and T2D over a six-year period (Jaziri *et al.* 2006). In normoglycaemic subjects at baseline, the risk of developing hyperglycaemia after six years was lower in subjects carrying the "12Ala" allele. Plasma insulin levels and HOMA-IR (insulin resistance index) were lower in subjects with the "Ala" allele compared to "Pro12Pro" subjects.

PPARsγ act at the nuclear level, as co-activators and co-repressors, i.e. they modulate gene transcription (Fig. 17) (Marion-Letellier *et al.* 2016). They are specifically expressed in white and brown adipose tissue, large intestine and spleen. However, their expression is highest in adipocytes and they play a key role in the regulation of adipogenesis, energy balance and lipid biosynthesis (Takada & Makishima 2020).

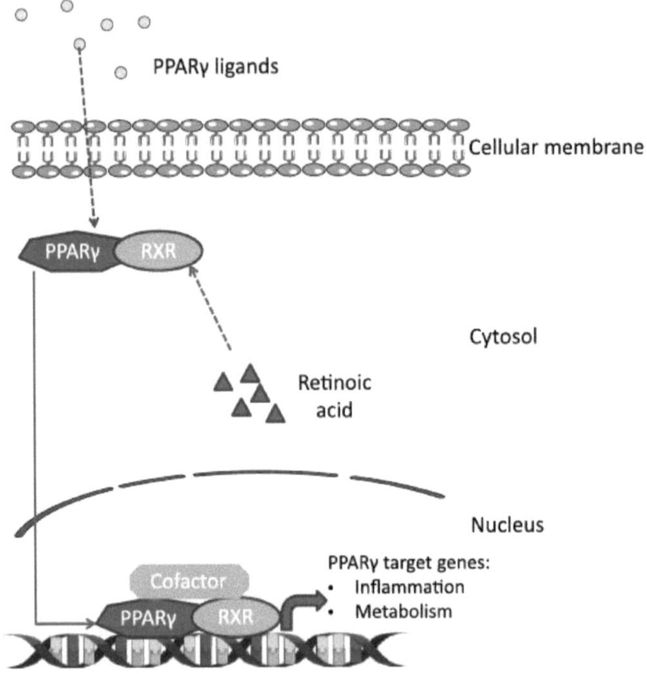

Figure 17: *PPAR* signalling pathwayγ. Adapted from (Marion-Letellier *et al.* 2016).

PPARγ is activated by many natural or synthetic ligands. After binding to a ligand, PPAR forms a heterodimer with the retinoid X receptor (RXR) which is activated by retinoic acid and recruits co-activators. The complex then binds to the peroxisome proliferator response element (PPRE) gene promoter, leading to the regulation of transcription of genes primarily involved in lipid and glucose metabolism, inflammation and cancer.

The role of *PPARγ* in T2DM is clearly suggested by the fact that thiazolidinediones (TZDs) improve the sensitivity of the insulin response. Many studies have shown that *PPARγ* is the molecular target of these pharmacological agents (Vallo *et al.* 2022). This is supported in particular by the fact that novel high-affinity *PPARγ* ligands strongly potentiate insulin sensitivity in vivo (Abbas *et al.* 2012; Mirza *et al.* 2019; Vallo *et al.* 2022). In fact, *PPARγ-related* reduction of insulin resistance occurs via regulation of key gene expression in the adipocyte (Gervois & Fruchart 2003) (Fig. 18). Thus, *PPARγ* promotes the flow of triglycerides to the adipose tissue, reserving the use of glucose by the brain, liver and muscle. Recently, many heterocyclic *PPAR* ligands have been developed for potential therapeutic applications (Virendra *et al.* 2022).

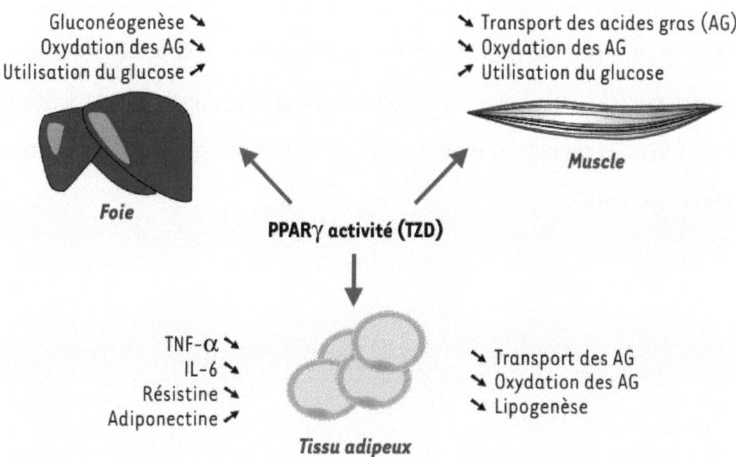

Figure 18: *PPARγ* improves insulin sensitivity. Adapted from (Gervois & Fruchart 2003).

Activation of PPARγ by thiazolidinediones promotes the flow of fatty acids and triglycerides to the adipose tissue. This results in a potentiation of glucose utilisation in the periphery. FA, fatty acids; TZD, thiazolidinediones.

5.3. *KCNJ11* and *ABCC8*

Sulphonylureas are the widely used oral agents for the treatment of T2DM, whose mechanism of action is the stimulation of insulin secretion via binding to the sulphonylurea receptor 1 (SUR1). ATP-sensitive potassium channels are important regulators of insulin secretion (Fig. 19). They consist of four SUR1 subunits (encoded by *ABCC8: ATP-binding cassette transporter subfamily C member 8*) and four Kir6.2 subunits (encoded by *KCNJ11: potassium inwardly-rectifying channel, subfamily J, member 11*).

The genes encoding Kir6.2 and SUR1 are located next to each other on human chromosome 11p15.1 (Fig. 20). Mutations in the *KCNJ11* or *ABCC8* genes could decrease or abolish the metabolic sensitivity of the K channel function$_{ATP}$ of pancreatic β cells, resulting in constant cell membrane depolarisation and persistent insulin secretion even at very low plasma glucose concentrations (Jahnavi *et al.* 2014).

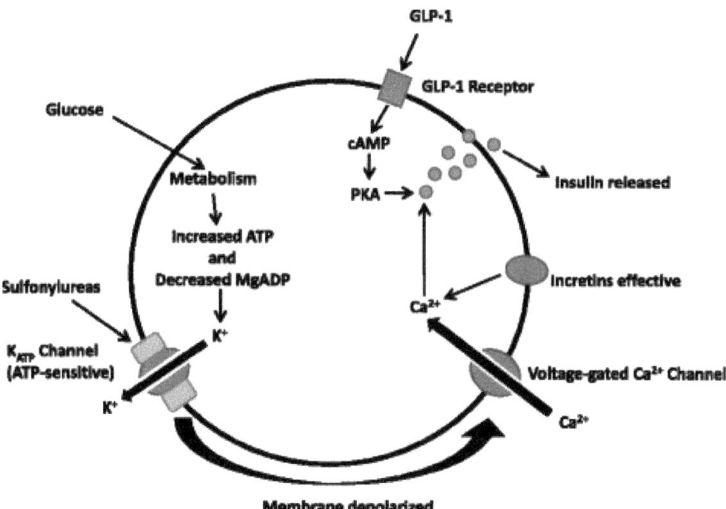

Figure 19: Molecular model of K-channel-mediated insulin secretion$_{ATP}$ comprising the *KCNJ11* and *ABCC8* subunits in the pancreatic β-cell. From (Song *et al.* 2017).

Intracellular glucose metabolism induces an increase in the ATP/ADP ratio which raises the degree of closure of ATP-sensitive membrane potassium (K^+) ion channels (K_{ATP} channels). This leads to the opening of voltage-dependent calcium channels and increases intracellular Ca^{2+}. A high cytosolic Ca^{2+} concentration triggers the fusion of insulin vesicles with the plasma membrane and insulin secretion. In addition, the interaction between sulphonylurea and its receptor (SUR1) causes inhibition of the K channel$_{ATP}$, a decrease in K efflux$^+$ and depolarisation of β-cells and by the same mechanism insulin secretion.

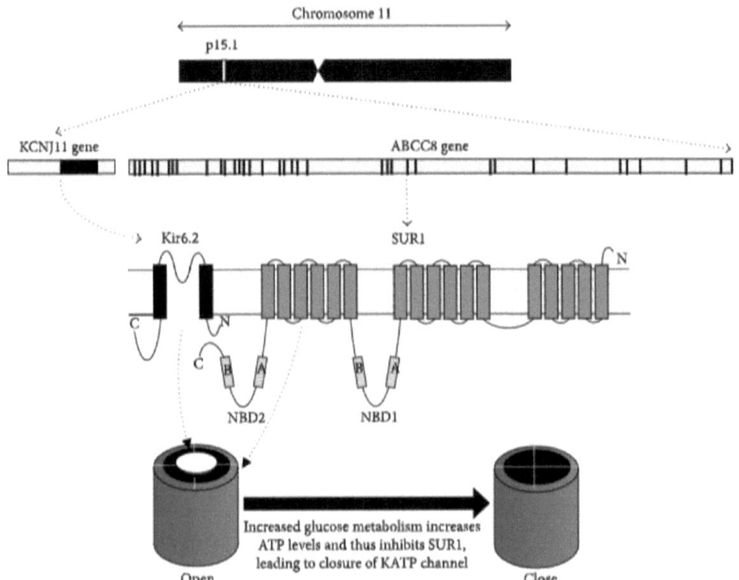

Figure 20: The genes encoding Kir6.2 (*KCNJ11*) and SUR1 (*ABCC8*) and their functions. From (Haghvirdizadeh *et al.* 2015).

The KCNJ11 and ABCC8 genes are located next to each other on human chromosome 11p15.1. Kir6.2: inward-rectifying potassium ion channel; SUR1: sulfonylurea receptor 1; NBD1: nucleotide-binding domain 1; NBD2: nucleotide-binding domain 2.

The *KCNJ11* gene encodes the Kir6.2 subunit of the K $channel_{ATP}$ of the pancreatic β-cell and other cell types. K $channels_{ATP}$ are particularly involved in the regulation of insulin secretion in response to changes in ATP levels in the pancreatic β-cell. Indeed, several studies have reported that the E23K polymorphism of KIR6.2 is accompanied by a discrete increase in susceptibility to T2DM (Gloyn *et al.* 2003; Florez *et al.* 2004; Cejková *et al.* 2007; Alsmadi *et al.* 2008; Lasram *et al.* 2014; Sokolova *et al.* 2015).

A recent global meta-analysis showed that the E23K variant of KIR6.2 is associated with an increased risk of T2D under the dominant genetic model (OR = 1.35 95% CI: 1.22 - 1.50; p<0.01). The recessive genetic model (OR = 0.78 95% CI: 0.67 - 0.91, $p<0.01$) was considered a protective factor for T2DM (Ren *et al.* 2022). In addition, a significant reduction in insulin secretion, decreased insulin concentrations and improved insulin sensitivity were shown to be related to the E23K variant of the *KCNJ11* gene (Villareal *et al.* 2009).

The S1369A variant (rs757110) located in exon 33 of the *ABCC8* gene is the most widely studied genetic polymorphism in sulphonylurea treatment in type 2 diabetes (Klen *et al.* 2014). Other polymorphisms have been investigated by several studies and are associated with an increased risk of T2DM (Haghverdizadeh *et al.* 2014).

Furthermore, the two variants E23K (*KCNJ11*) and S1369A (*ABCC8*) of the K $channel_{ATP}$, which are in strong binding disequilibrium, are found to form a haplotype that appears to be associated with a very high risk of T2DM (Fatehi *et al.* 2012).

Recently, mutations in the pancreatic β-cell potassium channel have been linked to permanent neonatal diabetes (Edghill *et al.* 2010; De Franco *et al.* 2020). Thus, *ABCC8/KCNJ11* variants should be suspected in children diagnosed with diabetes at less than 6 months of age, as in most of them the replacement of insulin by oral antidiabetic drugs is effective (Warncke *et al.* 2022).

5.4. *SLC30A8* and *IDE-KIF11-HHEX*

Two new variations located on the *SLC30A8* (Solute Carrier family 30, zinc transporter, member 8) gene and the cluster located on chromosome 10q23.33, which includes the *IDE* (insulin-degrading enzyme) gene, the *KIF11* (kinesin-interacting factor) gene and the *HHEX* (Hematopoietically Expressed Homeobox) gene, identified by a Franco-Canadian team, are associated with a higher risk of developing T2D (Sladek *et al.* 2007).

The *SLC30A8* gene produces the ZnT8 (zinc transporter member 8) protein which is involved in zinc transport. This transporter is expressed mainly in pancreatic β-cells and plays a key role in maintaining blood glucose concentration through its role in insulin storage, maturation and secretion (Chimienti *et al.* 2005; Davidson *et al.* 2014).

The *SLC30A8* gene is located on the long (q) arm of chromosome 8 at position 8q24.11. This gene is known by the existence of SNP rs13266634 in its last exon. In this SNP a change between the two C/T nucleotides occurs, leading to an alteration between the two amino acids arginine (R) and tryptophan (W) at position 325 (R325W). The R325 variant is characterised by a high efficiency in zinc transport and has been correlated with a higher risk of developing insulin resistance (Sala *et al.* 2021). In contrast, the W325 variant is less active and therefore plays a protective role against T2DM.

In a meta-analysis, Cheng *et al* (2015) show that their results suggest that the SNP rs13266634 is associated with an increased risk of T2D in Asian and European populations. This association is not demonstrated in the African population. In the Arab population, studies of the association of SNP rs13266634 with T2D are mixed. In Moroccan (Cauchi *et al.* 2008), Qatari (O'Beirne *et al.* 2016) and Lebanese (Mtiraoui *et al.* 2012) subjects, this SNP is not a risk factor for T2DM, whereas in the Jordanian (Mashal *et al.* 2021) and Tunisian (Turki *et al.* 2014) populations rs13266634 is associated with a risk of developing T2DM.

The *HHEX* gene encodes a transcription factor that is very important in pancreatic development (Foley & Mercola 2005). The *IDE* gene plays a key role in insulin degradation and in the initiation of cellular insulin processing (Tundo *et al.* 2017). It is located in the cell surface, cytosol, peroxisomes and endosomes of various insulin-sensitive tissues.

Results from a Chinese study confirm that genetic variants in the *IDE-KIF11-HHEX* region contribute to T2D susceptibility and suggest that the SNP rs7923837 may represent the strongest signal linked to T2D risk in the Chinese Han population (Qian *et al.* 2012).

5.5. *IGF2BP2, CDKN2A/B* and *CDKAL1*

In a spectacular collaboration, three groups from the whole genome studies (Diabetes Genetics Initiative 2007; Scott *et al.* 2007; Wellcome Trust Case Control Consortium 2007) joined forces (sample size 32554 individuals) to combine their initial findings. This collaboration led to the identification of new genes associated with T2DM: *IGF2BP2*, *CDKN2A/B* and *CDKAL1*.

The *IGF2BP2* (Insulin-like Growth Factor 2 mRNA Binding Protein 2) gene encodes a protein (BP2, Binding Protein 2) that binds to the IGF-2 transcript. As such, this protein regulates the translation of IGF-2 messenger RNA (Nielsen *et al.* 1999). IGF-2 is involved in cell proliferation and differentiation as well as in the stimulation of insulin action (Dai *et al.* 2020).

The *CDKN2B* (Cyclin-Dependent kinase inhibitor 2 B) and *CDKN2A* genes are located on chromosome 9p21 and code for the p15INK4b, P14ARF and p16INK4a proteins (Fig. 21).

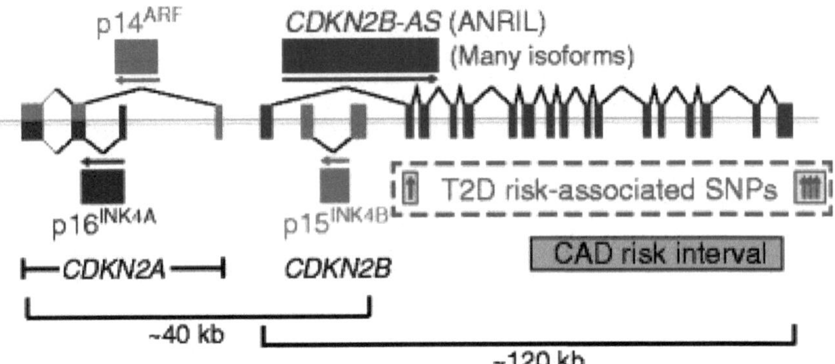

Figure 21: The human *CDKN2A/B* locus at chromosome 9p21. Adapted from (Kong *et al.* 2016).

*CDKN2A encodes both p16INK4A and p14ARF, which share exons 2 and 3. Polymorphisms influencing the risk of T2DM are distinct from the risk range for CAD (*Shea et al. 2011*). CAD, coronary heart disease*

The p16INK4a protein exerts its effect on β-cell replication by blocking the cyclin-dependent kinase 4 (CDK4) (Marzo *et al.* 2004). Studies in animal models have also demonstrated a major role for *CDKN2A* and *CDKN2B in* islet proliferation (Krishnamurthy *et al.* 2006). Polymorphisms in the *CDKN2A/B* genes are associated with the risk of T2D in various ethnicities including European, Asian, Indian, Mexican and Arab (Kong *et al.* 2016; Li *et al.* 2013).

Susceptibility to T2DM is also induced by the effect of variation in the *CDKAL1* gene [cyclin-dependent kinase 5 (CDK5) regulatory subunit associated protein 1-like 1] on reduced insulin secretion (Pascoe *et al.* 2008; Steinthorsdottir *et al.* 2007). This gene also affects the activity produced by the interaction of CDK5 with its receptor, which leads to the degeneration of pancreatic β-cells (Moore & Florez 2008). Steinthorsdottir et al. found that insulin response is decreased by 22% in homozygotes compared to heterozygotes and non-carriers of the mutation (Steinthorsdottir *et al.* 2007). The *CDKAL1* gene SNPs most associated with T2DM are rs7756992, rs7754840 and rs10946398 (Dehwah *et al.* 2010).

Recent studies have highlighted that variations in the *CDKAL1* gene transcript are responsible for the accumulation of misreplicated insulin and thus generate oxidative stress in pancreatic β-cells, leading to their destruction (Ghosh *et al.* 2022).

5.6. *ENPP1: A common gene for obesity and T2D*

ENPP1 (Ectonucleotidase Pyrophosphatase Phosphodiesterase 1), also known as PC-1 (Plasma Cell Membrane Glycoprotein 1), is a transmembrane glycoprotein that produces inorganic pyrophosphate, a major inhibitor of calcification and mineralisation (Bacci *et al.* 2007). *ENPP1* has been described as an inhibitor of the insulin receptor in fibroblasts from insulin-resistant and diabetic patients (Maddux *et al.* 2006). Inhibition of the tyrosine kinase activity of the insulin receptor is thought to occur through direct interaction of *ENPP1* with the α-subunit and inhibits the autophosphorylation of the receptor required for signal transduction (Maddux & Goldfine 2000). *ENPP1* is expressed in plasma, placenta, kidney, chondrocytes, but also in muscle, adipose tissue and liver, three key organs in the insulin response (Abate *et al.* 2006). *ENPP1* expression is involved in the maturation of adipose tissue. Thus, their interaction with the insulin receptor not only induces a failure in insulin signalling but also a failure in adipocyte maturation (Liang *et al.* 2007).

Many studies have shown a significant association between the Q allele of the K121Q mutation of the *ENPP1* gene and the risk of T2D and insulin resistance (Fajar 2016). It should be noted that this association has not been found in many recent studies (Lyon *et al.* 2006; Keshavarz *et al.* 2006; Weedon *et al.* 2006; Zhao *et al.* 2011; Saberi *et al.* 2011), especially in a Danish population of 7,333 individuals (Grarup *et al.* 2006). In the same study, a meta-analysis of Danish populations and other previous studies found a significant association between the Q121 allele and the risk of T2DM. In another meta-analysis of 42,042 individuals (*ENPP1* Consortium), McAteer et al. found that the Q121 variant increases the risk of developing T2D under the recessive model in European descendants (OR = 1.38 [95% CI 1.10-1.74] p = 0.005) and is modulated by BMI (McAteer *et al.* 2008).

On the other hand, several studies have highlighted the modulating effect of the Q121 allele of the *ENPP1* gene in obesity risk (Meyre *et al.* 2007; Grarup *et al.* 2006; Matsuoka *et al.* 2006; McAteer *et al.* 2008; El Achhab *et al.* 2009; Zhao *et al.* 2011). Among these studies, some found a positive association between the Q121 allele and increased BMI, while others found the opposite. In other studies, the variant has no effect on BMI (Grarup *et al.* 2006; Lyon *et al.* 2006; Weedon *et al.* 2006; Zhao *et al.* 2011).

The discrepancy in association studies may be due to the wide variation in the frequency of this variant according to the ethnic origin of the populations studied. Indeed, this frequency is estimated at 77.3% in African Americans, 16.7% in European Americans, 10.5% in Japanese and 4.2% in Chinese

(Keshavarz *et al.* 2006). The recruitment procedures adopted by the studies may also play a role.

These data suggest the importance of insulin signal transduction molecules in susceptibility to metabolic diseases and their crucial role in maintaining normal insulin sensitivity.

References

Abate, N., Chandalia, M., Di Paola, R., Foster, D. W., Grundy, S. M., & Trischitta, V. (2006). Mechanisms of disease: Ectonucleotide pyrophosphatase phosphodiesterase 1 as a 'gatekeeper' of insulin receptors. *Nature Clinical Practice Endocrinology & Metabolism*, 2(12), 694-701.

Abbas, A., Blandon, J., Rude, J., Elfar, A., & Mukherjee, D. (2012). PPAR-γ agonist in treatment of diabetes: cardiovascular safety considerations. *Cardiovascular & Hematological Agents in Medicinal Chemistry (Formerly Current Medicinal Chemistry-Cardiovascular & Hematological Agents)*, 10(2), 124-134.

Alsmadi, O., Al-Rubeaan, K., Wakil, S. M., Imtiaz, F., Mohamed, G., Al-Saud, H., ... & Meyer, B. F. (2008). Genetic study of Saudi diabetes (GSSD): significant association of the KCNJ11 E23K polymorphism with type 2 diabetes. *Diabetes/metabolism research and reviews*, 24(2), 137-140.

Al-Samarai, F. R., & Al-Kazaz, A. A. (2015). Molecular markers: An introduction and applications. *European journal of molecular biotechnology*, 9(3), 118-130.

Avise, J. C. (2012). *Molecular markers, natural history and evolution*. Springer Science & Business Media.

Bacci, S., De Cosmo, S., Prudente, S., & Trischitta, V. (2007). ENPP1 gene, insulin resistance and related clinical outcomes. *Current Opinion in Clinical Nutrition & Metabolic Care*, 10(4), 403-409.

Ballinger, S. W., Shoffner, J. M., Hedaya, E. V., Trounce, I., Polak, M. A., Koontz, D. A., & Wallace, D. C. (1992). Maternally transmitted diabetes and deafness associated with a 10.4 kb mitochondrial DNA deletion. *Nature genetics*, 1(1), 11-15.

Barroso, I. (2005). Genetics of type 2 diabetes. *Diabetic medicine*, 22(5), 517-535.

Bell, C. G., Walley, A. J., & Froguel, P. (2005). The genetics of human obesity. *Nature reviews genetics*, 6(3), 221-234.

Blackwelder, W. C., Elston, R. C., & Rao, D. C. (1985). A comparison of sib-pair linkage tests for disease susceptibility loci. *Genetic Epidemiology*, 2(1), 85-97.

Bodhini, D., Radha, V., Dhar, M., Narayani, N., & Mohan, V. (2007). The rs12255372 (G/T) and rs7903146 (C/T) polymorphisms of the TCF7L2 gene are associated with type 2 diabetes mellitus in Asian Indians. *Metabolism*, 56(9), 1174-1178.

Botstein, D., White, R. L., Skolnick, M., & Davis, R. W. (1980). Construction of a genetic linkage map in man using restriction fragment length polymorphisms. *American journal of human genetics*, 32(3), 314.

Cardon, L. R., & Palmer, L. J. (2003). Population stratification and spurious allelic association. *The Lancet*, 361(9357), 598-604.

Carulli, L., Rondinella, S., Lombardini, S., Canedi, I., Loria, P., & Carulli, N. (2005). Diabetes, genetics and ethnicity. *Alimentary pharmacology & therapeutics*, 22, 16-19.

Cauchi, S., Meyre, D., Dina, C., Choquet, H., Samson, C., Gallina, S., ... & Froguel, P. (2006). Transcription factor TCF7L2 genetic study in the French population: expression in human β-cells and adipose tissue and strong association with type 2 diabetes. *Diabetes*, 55(10), 2903-2908.

Cauchi, S., Meyre, D., Durand, E., Proença, C., Marre, M., Hadjadj, S., ... & Froguel, P. (2008). Post genome-wide association studies of novel genes associated with type 2 diabetes show gene-gene interaction and high predictive value. *PloS one*, 3(5), e2031.

Cauchi, S., El Achhab, Y., Choquet, H., Dina, C., Krempler, F., Weitgasser, R., ... & Froguel, P. (2007). TCF7L2 is reproducibly associated with type 2 diabetes in various ethnic groups: a global meta-analysis. *Journal of molecular medicine*, 85(7), 777-782.

Čejková, P., Novota, P., Černá, M., Kološtová, K., Nováková, D., Kučera, P., ... & Ždárský, E. (2007). KCNJ11 E23K polymorphism and diabetes mellitus with adult onset in Czech patients. *Folia Biologica (Praha)*, 53, 173-175.

Chang, H. W., Chuang, L. Y., Cheng, Y. H., Ho, C. H., Wen, C. H., & Yang, C. H. (2009). Seq-SNPing: multiple-alignment tool for SNP discovery, SNP ID identification, and RFLP genotyping. *OMICS A Journal of Integrative Biology*, 13(3), 253-260.

Chen, J., Ning, C., Mu, J., Li, D., Ma, Y., & Meng, X. (2021). Role of Wnt signaling pathways in type 2 diabetes mellitus. *Molecular and Cellular Biochemistry*, 476(5), 2219-2232.

Cheng, L., Zhang, D., Zhou, L., Zhao, J., & Chen, B. (2015). Association between SLC30A8 rs13266634 polymorphism and type 2 diabetes risk: a meta-analysis. *Medical science monitor: international medical journal of experimental and clinical research*, 21, 2178.

Chimienti, F., Favier, A., & Seve, M. (2005). ZnT-8, a pancreatic beta-cell-specific zinc transporter. *Biometals*, 18(4), 313-317.

Choi, S. W., Mak, T. S. H., & O'Reilly, P. F. (2020). Tutorial: a guide to performing polygenic risk score analyses. *Nature protocols*, 15(9), 2759-2772.

Colhoun, H. M., McKeigue, P. M., & Smith, G. D. (2003). Problems of reporting genetic associations with complex outcomes. *The Lancet*, 361(9360), 865-872.

Cordell, H. J., & Clayton, D. G. (2005). Genetic association studies. *The Lancet*, 366(9491), 1121-1131.

Crawford, D. C., & Nickerson, D. A. (2005). Definition and clinical importance of haplotypes. *Annual review of medicine*, 56, 303.

Dai, N. (2020). The diverse functions of IMP2/IGF2BP2 in metabolism. *Trends in Endocrinology & Metabolism*, 31(9), 670-679.

Davidson, H. W., Wenzlau, J. M., & O'Brien, R. M. (2014). Zinc transporter 8 (ZnT8) and β cell function. *Trends in Endocrinology & Metabolism*, 25(8), 415-424.

De Franco, E., Saint-Martin, C., Brusgaard, K., Knight Johnson, A. E., Aguilar-Bryan, L., Bowman, P., ... & Flanagan, S. E. (2020). Update of variants identified in the pancreatic β-cell KATP channel genes KCNJ11 and ABCC8 in individuals with congenital hyperinsulinism and diabetes. *Human mutation*, 41(5), 884-905.

Deeb, S. S., Fajas, L., Nemoto, M., Pihlajamäki, J., Mykkänen, L., Kuusisto, J., ... & Auwerx, J. (1998). A Pro12Ala substitution in PPARγ2 associated with decreased receptor activity, lower body mass index and improved insulin sensitivity. *Nature genetics*, 20(3), 284-287.

Dehwah, M. A., Wang, M., & Huang, Q. Y. (2010). CDKAL1 and type 2 diabetes: a global meta-analysis. *Genet Mol Res*, 9(2), 1109-1120.

del Bosque-Plata, L., Hernández-Cortés, E. P., & Gragnoli, C. (2022). The broad pathogenetic role of TCF7L2 in human diseases beyond type 2 diabetes. *Journal of Cellular Physiology*, 237(1), 301-312.

del Bosque-Plata, L., Martínez-Martínez, E., Espinoza-Camacho, M. Á., & Gragnoli, C. (2021). The role of TCF7L2 in type 2 diabetes. *Diabetes*, 70(6), 1220-1228.

Dheur, S., & Saupe, S. J. (2020). Genome-wide polygenic scores as a new form of human measurement. *History and Distemper Bulletin of the Life Sciences*, 27(1), 67-83.

Dornbos, P., Raffield, L., Yin, X., & Flannick, J. (2020). 241-OR: Causal Gene Candidates for Type 2 Diabetes Based on Protein-Coding Variants in 127,676 Individuals. *Diabetes*, 69(Supplement_1).

Duval, A., Rolland, S., Tubacher, E., Bui, H., Thomas, G., & Hamelin, R. (2000). The human T-cell transcription factor-4 gene: structure, extensive characterization of alternative splicings, and mutational analysis in colorectal cancer cell lines. *Cancer research*, 60(14), 3872-3879.

Eaves, I. A., Bennett, S. T., Forster, P., Ferber, K. M., Ehrmann, D., Wilson, A. J., ... & Todd, J. A. (1999). Transmission ratio distortion at the INS-IGF2 VNTR. *Nature genetics*, 22(4), 324-325.

Edghill, E. L., Flanagan, S. E., & Ellard, S. (2010). Permanent neonatal diabetes due to activating mutations in ABCC8 and KCNJ11. *Reviews in endocrine and metabolic disorders*, 11(3), 193-198.

El Achhab, Y., Meyre, D., Bouatia-Naji, N., Berraho, M., Deweirder, M., Vatin, V., ... & Chikri, M. (2009). Association of the ENPP1 K121Q polymorphism with type 2 diabetes and obesity in the Moroccan population. *Diabetes & metabolism*, 35(1), 37-42.

Ellegren, H. (2004). Microsatellites: simple sequences with complex evolution. *Nature reviews genetics*, 5(6), 435-445.

Evans, D. M., & Cardon, L. R. (2004). Guidelines for genotyping in genomewide linkage studies: single-nucleotide-polymorphism maps versus microsatellite maps. *The American Journal of Human Genetics*, 75(4), 687-692.

Fajar, J. K. (2016). The association of ectonucleotide pyrophosphatase/phosphodiesterase 1 (ENPP1) K121Q gene polymorphism with the risk of type 2 diabetes mellitus in European, American, and African populations: A meta-analysis. *Journal of Health Sciences*, 6(2), 76-86.

Fatehi, M., Raja, M., Carter, C., Soliman, D., Holt, A., & Light, P. E. (2012). The ATP-sensitive K+ channel ABCC8 S1369A type 2 diabetes risk variant increases MgATPase activity. *Diabetes*, 61(1), 241-249.

Florez, J. C., Burtt, N., De Bakker, P. I., Almgren, P., Tuomi, T., Holmkvist, J., ... & Altshuler, D. (2004). Haplotype structure and genotype-phenotype correlations of the sulfonylurea receptor and the islet ATP-sensitive potassium channel gene region. *Diabetes*, 53(5), 1360-1368.

Florez, J. C., Jablonski, K. A., Bayley, N., Pollin, T. I., de Bakker, P. I., Shuldiner, A. R., ... & Altshuler, D. (2006). TCF7L2 polymorphisms and progression to diabetes in the Diabetes Prevention Program. *New England Journal of Medicine*, 355(3), 241-250.

Foley, A. C., & Mercola, M. (2005). Heart induction by Wnt antagonists depends on the homeodomain transcription factor Hex. *Genes & development*, 19(3), 387-396.

Franks, P. W., Mesa, J. L., Harding, A. H., & Wareham, N. J. (2007). Gene-lifestyle interaction on risk of type 2 diabetes. *Nutrition, metabolism and cardiovascular diseases*, 17(2), 104-124.

Ge, T., Irvin, M. R., Patki, A., Srinivasasainagendra, V., Lin, Y. F., Tiwari, H. K., ... & Karlson, E. W. (2022). Development and validation of a trans-ancestry polygenic risk score for type 2 diabetes in diverse populations. *Genome medicine*, 14(1), 1-16.

Gervois, P., & Fruchart, J. C. (2003). PPARγ: a major nuclear receptor in adipogenesis. *M/S: medicine sciences*, 19(1), 20-22.

Ghosh, C., Das, N., Saha, S., Kundu, T., Sircar, D., & Roy, P. (2022). Involvement of Cdkal1 in the etiology of type 2 diabetes mellitus and microvascular diabetic complications: a review. *Journal of Diabetes & Metabolic Disorders*, 1-11.

Gloyn, A. L., Weedon, M. N., Owen, K. R., Turner, M. J., Knight, B. A., Hitman, G., ... & Frayling, T. M. (2003). Large-scale association studies of variants in genes encoding the pancreatic β-cell KATP channel subunits Kir6. 2 (KCNJ11) and SUR1 (ABCC8) confirm that the KCNJ11 E23K variant is associated with type 2 diabetes. *Diabetes*, 52(2), 568-572.

Gouda, H. N., Sagoo, G. S., Harding, A. H., Yates, J., Sandhu, M. S., & Higgins, J. P. (2010). The association between the peroxisome proliferator-activated receptor-γ2 (PPARG2) Pro12Ala gene variant and type 2 diabetes mellitus: a HuGE review and meta-analysis. *American journal of epidemiology*, 171(6), 645-655.

Grant, S. F. (2019). The TCF7L2 locus: a genetic window into the pathogenesis of type 1 and type 2 diabetes. *Diabetes Care*, 42(9), 1624-1629.

Grant, S. F., Thorleifsson, G., Reynisdottir, I., Benediktsson, R., Manolescu, A., Sainz, J., ... & Stefansson, K. (2006). Variant of transcription factor 7-like 2 (TCF7L2) gene confers risk of type 2 diabetes. *Nature genetics*, 38(3), 320-323.

Grarup, N., & Andersen, G. (2007). Gene-environment interactions in the pathogenesis of type 2 diabetes and metabolism. *Current Opinion in Clinical Nutrition & Metabolic Care*, 10(4), 420-426.

Grarup, N., Urhammer, S. A., Ek, J., Albrechtsen, A., Glümer, C., Borch-Johnsen, K., ... & Pedersen, O. (2006). Studies of the relationship between the ENPP1 K121Q polymorphism and type 2 diabetes, insulin resistance and obesity in 7,333 Danish white subjects. *Diabetologia*, 49, 2097-2104.

Groop, L. C., & Tuomi, T. (1997). Non-insulin-dependent diabetes mellitus-a collision between thrifty genes and an affluent society. *Annals of medicine*, 29(1), 37-53.

Guinan, K., Beauchemin, C., Tremblay, J., Chalmers, J., Woodward, M., Tahir, M. R., ... & Lachaine, J. (2021). Economic evaluation of a new polygenic risk score to predict nephropathy in adult patients with type 2 diabetes. *Canadian Journal of Diabetes*, 45(2), 129-136.

Haghverdizadeh, P., Haerian, M. S., Haghverdizadeh, P., & Haerian, B. S. (2014). ABCC8 genetic variants and risk of diabetes mellitus. *Gene*, 545(2), 198-204.

Haghvirdizadeh, P., Mohamed, Z., Abdullah, N. A., Haghvirdizadeh, P., Haerian, M. S., & Haerian, B. S. (2015). KCNJ11: genetic polymorphisms and risk of diabetes mellitus. *Journal of diabetes research, 2015*.

Healy, D. G. (2006). Case-control studies in the genomic era: a clinician's guide. *The Lancet Neurology*, 5(8), 701-707.

Hirschhorn, J. N., & Daly, M. J. (2005). Genome-wide association studies for common diseases and complex traits. *Nature reviews genetics*, 6(2), 95-108.

Horvath, S., & Laird, N. M. (1998). A discordant-sibship test for disequilibrium and linkage: no need for parental data. *The American Journal of Human Genetics*, 63(6), 1886-1897.

Hu, F. B., & Willett, W. C. (2001). Diet and coronary heart disease: findings from the Nurses' Health Study and Health Professionals' Follow-up Study. *The journal of nutrition, health & aging*, 5(3), 132-138.

Hunter, D. J. (2005). Gene-environment interactions in human diseases. *Nature reviews genetics*, 6(4), 287-298.

Jahnavi, S., Poovazhagi, V., Kanthimathi, S., Balamurugan, K., Bodhini, D., Yadav, J., ... & Radha, V. (2014). Novel ABCC8 (SUR1) gene mutations in Asian Indian children with congenital hyperinsulinemic hypoglycemia. *Annals of human genetics*, 78(5), 311-319.

Jaziri, R., Lobbens, S., Aubert, R., Péan, F., Lahmidi, S., Vaxillaire, M., ... & DESIR Study Group (2006). The PPARG Pro12Ala polymorphism is associated with a decreased risk of developing hyperglycemia over 6 years and combines with the effect of the APM1 G-11391A single nucleotide polymorphism: the Data From an Epidemiological Study on the Insulin Resistance Syndrome (DESIR) study. *Diabetes*, 55(4), 1157-1162.

Keshavarz, P., Inoue, H., Sakamoto, Y., Kunika, K., Tanahashi, T., Nakamura, N., ... & Itakura, M. (2006). No evidence for association of the ENPP1 (PC-1) K121Q variant with risk of type 2 diabetes in a Japanese population. *Journal of human genetics*, 51, 559-566.

Kim, S., & Misra, A. (2007). SNP genotyping: technologies and biomedical applications. *Annu. Rev. Biomed. Eng*, 9, 289-320.

King H, Rewers M (1993) Global estimates for prevalence of diabetes mellitus and impaired glucose tolerance in adults. WHO Ad Hoc Diabetes Reporting Group. *Diabetes Care* 16:157-77.

Klen, J., Dolžan, V., & Janež, A. (2014). CYP2C9, KCNJ11 and ABCC8 polymorphisms and the response to sulphonylurea treatment in type 2 diabetes patients. *European journal of clinical pharmacology*, 70(4), 421-428.

Knop, M. R., Geng, T. T., Gorny, A. W., Ding, R., Li, C., Ley, S. H., & Huang, T. (2018). Birth weight and risk of type 2 diabetes mellitus, cardiovascular disease, and hypertension in adults: a meta-analysis of 7 646 267 participants from 135 studies. *Journal of the American Heart Association*, 7(23), e008870.

Knowler, W. C., Pettitt, D. J., Saad, M. F., & Bennett, P. H. (1990). Diabetes mellitus in the Pima Indians: incidence, risk factors and pathogenesis. *Diabetes/metabolism reviews*, 6(1), 1-27.

Kolb, H., & Martin, S. (2017). Environmental/lifestyle factors in the pathogenesis and prevention of type 2 diabetes. *BMC medicine*, 15(1), 1-11.

Kong, Y., Sharma, R. B., Nwosu, B. U., & Alonso, L. C. (2016). Islet biology, the CDKN2A/B locus and type 2 diabetes risk. *Diabetologia*, 59(8), 1579-1593.

Krishnamurthy, J., Ramsey, M. R., Ligon, K. L., Torrice, C., Koh, A., Bonner-Weir, S., & Sharpless, N. E. (2006). p16INK4a induces an age-dependent decline in islet regenerative potential. *Nature*, 443(7110), 453-457.

Ktorza, A., Bernard, C., Parent, V., Pénicaud, L., Froguel, P., Lathrop, M., & Gauguier, D. (1997). Are animal models of diabetes relevant to the study of the genetics of non-insulin-dependent diabetes in humans? *Diabetes & metabolism*, 23, 38-46.

Laird, N. M., & Lange, C. (2006). Family-based designs in the age of large-scale gene-association studies. *Nature Reviews Genetics*, 7(5), 385-394.

Lasram, K., Ben Halim, N., Hsouna, S., Kefi, R., Arfa, I., Ghazouani, W., ... & Abdelhak, S. (2014). Evidence for association of the E23K variant of KCNJ11 gene with type 2 diabetes in

Tunisian population: population-based study and meta-analysis. *BioMed Research International*, 2014.

Le Bacquer, O., Shu, L., Marchand, M., Neve, B., Paroni, F., Kerr Conte, J., ... & Maedler, K. (2011). TCF7L2 splice variants have distinct effects on β-cell turnover and function. *Human molecular genetics*, 20(10), 1906-1915.

Li, H., Tang, X., Liu, Q., & Wang, Y. (2013). Association between type 2 diabetes and rs10811661 polymorphism upstream of CDKN2A/B: a meta-analysis. *Acta diabetologica*, 50(5), 657-662.

Liang, J., Fu, M., Ciociola, E., Chandalia, M., & Abate, N. (2007). Role of ENPP1 on adipocyte maturation. *PLoS one*, 2(9), e882.

Little, J., Higgins, J. P., Ioannidis, J. P., Moher, D., Gagnon, F., Von Elm, E., ... & Birkett, N. (2009). STrengthening the REporting of Genetic Association Studies (STREGA) - an extension of the STROBE statement. *Genetic Epidemiology: The Official Publication of the International Genetic Epidemiology Society*, 33(7), 581-598.

Lyon, H. N., Florez, J. C., Bersaglieri, T., Saxena, R., Winckler, W., Almgren, P., ... & Hirschhorn, J. N. (2006). Common variants in the ENPP1 gene are not reproducibly associated with diabetes or obesity. *diabetes*, 55(11), 3180-3184.

Lyssenko, V., Lupi, R., Marchetti, P., Del Guerra, S., Orho-Melander, M., Almgren, P., ... & Groop, L. (2007). Mechanisms by which common variants in the TCF7L2 gene increase risk of type 2 diabetes. *The Journal of clinical investigation*, 117(8), 2155-2163.

Lander, E. S., & Schork, N. J. (2006). Genetic dissection of complex traits. *FOCUS*, 265(3), 2037-458.

Li, M., Rivière, J. B., & Polychronakos, C. (2021). Why all MODY variants are dominantly inherited: a hypothesis. *Trends in Genetics*.

Maassen, J. A., Janssen, G. M., & Hart, L. M. (2005). Molecular mechanisms of mitochondrial diabetes (MIDD). *Annals of medicine*, 37(3), 213-221.

Maddux, B. A., Chang, Y. N., Accili, D., McGuinness, O. P., Youngren, J. F., & Goldfine, I. D. (2006). Overexpression of the insulin receptor inhibitor PC-1/ENPP1 induces insulin resistance and hyperglycemia. *American Journal of Physiology-Endocrinology and Metabolism*, 290(4), E746-E749.

Maddux, B. A., & Goldfine, I. D. (2000). Membrane glycoprotein PC-1 inhibition of insulin receptor function occurs via direct interaction with the receptor alpha-subunit. *Diabetes*, 49(1), 13-19.

Mahajan, A., Spracklen, C. N., Zhang, W., Ng, M. C., Petty, L. E., Kitajima, H., ... & Jørgensen, M. E. (2022). Multi-ancestry genetic study of type 2 diabetes highlights the power of diverse populations for discovery and translation. *Nature Genetics*, 54(5), 560-572.

Marion-Letellier, R., Savoye, G., & Ghosh, S. (2016). Fatty acids, eicosanoids and PPAR gamma. *European journal of pharmacology*, *785*, 44-49.

Mars, N., Kerminen, S., Feng, Y. C. A., Kanai, M., Läll, K., Thomas, L. F., ... & Biobank Japan Project (2022). Genome-wide risk prediction of common diseases across ancestries in one million people. *Cell genomics*, 2(4), 100118.

Marzo, N., Mora, C., Fabregat, M. E., Martin, J., Usac, E. F., Franco, C., ... & Gomis, R. (2004). Pancreatic islets from cyclin-dependent kinase 4/R24C (Cdk4) knockin mice have significantly increased beta cell mass and are physiologically functional, indicating that Cdk4 is a potential target for pancreatic beta cell mass regeneration in Type 1 diabetes. *Diabetologia*, 47(4), 686-694.

Mashal, S., Khanfar, M., Al-Khalayfa, S., Srour, L., Mustafa, L., Hakooz, N. M., ... & Azab, B. (2021). SLC30A8 gene polymorphism rs13266634 associated with increased risk for developing type 2 diabetes mellitus in Jordanian population. *Gene*, *768*, 145279.

Matsuoka, N., Patki, A., Tiwari, H. K., Allison, D. B., Johnson, S. B., Gregersen, P. K., ... & Chung, W. K. (2006). Association of K121Q polymorphism in ENPP1 (PC-1) with BMI in Caucasian and African-American adults. *International journal of obesity*, *30*(2), 233-237.

Mayeux, R. (2005). Mapping the new frontier: complex genetic disorders. *The Journal of clinical investigation*, 115(6), 1404-1407.

McAteer, J. B., Prudente, S., Bacci, S., Lyon, H. N., Hirschhorn, J. N., Trischitta, V., ... & ENPP1 Consortium (2008). The ENPP1 K121Q polymorphism is associated with type 2 diabetes in European populations: evidence from an updated meta-analysis in 42,042 subjects. *Diabetes*, 57(4), 1125-1130.

Meigs, J. B. (2019). The genetic epidemiology of type 2 diabetes: opportunities for health translation. *Current diabetes reports*, 19(8), 1-8.

Meigs, J. B., Cupples, L. A., & Wilson, P. W. (2000). Parental transmission of type 2 diabetes: the Framingham Offspring Study. *Diabetes*, 49(12), 2201-2207.

Meyer, B. F., Alsmadi, O., Wakil, S., & Al-Rubeaan, K. (2009). Genetics of type 2 diabetes in Arabs: What we know to date. *International Journal of Diabetes Mellitus*, 1(1), 32-34.

Meyre, D., Bouatia-Naji, N., Vatin, V., Veslot, J., Samson, C., Tichet, J., ... & Froguel, P. (2007). ENPP1 K121Q polymorphism and obesity, hyperglycaemia and type 2 diabetes in the prospective DESIR Study. *Diabetologia*, 50, 2090-2096.

Mirza, A. Z., Althagafi, I. I., & Shamshad, H. (2019). Role of PPAR receptor in different diseases and their ligands: Physiological importance and clinical implications. *European Journal of Medicinal Chemistry*, 166, 502-513.

Miyake, K., Horikawa, Y., Hara, K., Yasuda, K., Osawa, H., Furuta, H., ... & Kasuga, M. (2008). Association of TCF7L2 polymorphisms with susceptibility to type 2 diabetes in 4,087 Japanese subjects. *Journal of human genetics*, 53(2), 174-180.

Moore, A. F., & Florez, J. C. (2008). Genetic susceptibility to type 2 diabetes and implications for antidiabetic therapy. *Annu. Rev Med* 59, 95-111.

Mtiraoui, N., Turki, A., Nemr, R., Echtay, A., Izzidi, I., Al-Zaben, G. S., ... & Almawi, W. Y. (2012). Contribution of common variants of ENPP1, IGF2BP2, KCNJ11, MLXIPL, PPARγ, SLC30A8 and TCF7L2 to the risk of type 2 diabetes in Lebanese and Tunisian Arabs. *Diabetes & metabolism*, 38(5), 444-449.

Nachtomy, O., Shavit, A., & Yakhini, Z. (2007). Gene expression and the concept of the phenotype. *Studies in History and Philosophy of Science Part C: Studies in History and Philosophy of Biological and Biomedical Sciences*, 38(1), 238-254.

Neel, J. V. (1962). Diabetes mellitus: a "thrifty" genotype rendered detrimental by "progress"? *American journal of human genetics*, 14(4), 353.

Newman, B. J. M. C. R. G., Selby, J. V., King, M. C., Slemenda, C., Fabsitz, R., & Friedman, G. D. (1987). Concordance for type 2 (non-insulin-dependent) diabetes mellitus in male twins. *Diabetologia*, 30(10), 763-768.

Nielsen, J., Christiansen, J., Lykke-Andersen, J., Johnsen, A. H., Wewer, U. M., & Nielsen, F. C. (1999). A family of insulin-like growth factor II mRNA-binding proteins represses translation in late development. *Molecular and cellular biology*, 19(2), 1262-1270.

O'Beirne, S. L., Salit, J., Rodriguez-Flores, J. L., Staudt, M. R., Abi Khalil, C., Fakhro, K. A., ... & Crystal, R. G. (2016). Type 2 diabetes risk allele loci in the Qatari population. *PloS one*, 11(7), e0156834.

Osawa, H., Yamada, K., Onuma, H., Murakami, A., Ochi, M., Kawata, H., ... & Makino, H. (2004). The G/G genotype of a resistin single-nucleotide polymorphism at- 420 increases type 2 diabetes mellitus susceptibility by inducing promoter activity through specific binding of Sp1/3. *The American Journal of Human Genetics*, 75(4), 678-686.

Pai, T. W., & Chen, C. M. (2016). SSRs as genetic markers in the human genome and their observable relationship to hereditary diseases. *Biomarkers in Medicine*, 10(6), 563-566.

Pascoe, L., Frayling, T. M., Weedon, M. N., Mari, A., Tura, A., Ferrannini, E., ... & RISC Consortium (2008). Beta cell glucose sensitivity is decreased by 39% in non-diabetic individuals carrying multiple diabetes-risk alleles compared with those with no risk alleles. *Diabetologia*, 51, 1989-1992.

Permutt, M. A., Wasson, J., & Cox, N. (2005). Genetic epidemiology of diabetes. *The Journal of clinical investigation*, 115(6), 1431-1439.

Poulsen, P., Ohm Kyvik, K., Vaag, A., & Beck-Nielsen, H. (1999). Heritability of type II (non-insulin-dependent) diabetes mellitus and abnormal glucose tolerance-a population-based twin study. *Diabetologia*, 42(2), 139-145.

Qi, L., Van Dam, R. M., Asselbergs, F. W., & Hu, F. B. (2007). Gene-gene interactions between HNF4A and KCNJ11 in predicting Type 2 diabetes in women. *Diabetic Medicine*, 24(11), 1187-1191.

Qian, Y., Lu, F., Dong, M., Lin, Y., Li, H., Chen, J., ... & Shen, H. (2012). Genetic variants of IDE-KIF11-HHEX at 10q23.33 associated with type 2 diabetes risk: a fine-mapping study in Chinese population. *PloS one*, 7(4), e35060.

Rao, D. C. (2001). 3 Genetic dissection of complex traits: An overview. *Advances in Genetics*, 42, 13-34.

Redden, D. T., & Allison, D. B. (2003). Nonreplication in genetic association studies of obesity and diabetes research. *The Journal of nutrition*, 133(11), 3323-3326.

Ren, Y., Zhu, W., Shi, J., Shao, A., Cheng, Y., & Liu, Y. (2022). Association between KCNJ11 E23K polymorphism and the risk of type 2 diabetes mellitus: A global meta-analysis. *Journal of Diabetes and its Complications*, 36(5), 108170.

Saadi, H., Nagelkerke, N., Carruthers, S. G., Benedict, S., Abdulkhalek, S., Reed, R., ... & Nicholls, M. G. (2008). Association of TCF7L2 polymorphism with diabetes mellitus, metabolic syndrome, and markers of beta cell function and insulin resistance in a population-based sample of Emirati subjects. *Diabetes research and clinical practice*, 80(3), 392-398.

Saberi, H., Mohammadtaghvaei, N., Gulkho, S., Bakhtiyari, S., Mohammadi, M., Hanachi, P., ... & Meshkani, R. (2011). The ENPP1 K121Q polymorphism is not associated with type 2 diabetes and related metabolic traits in an Iranian population. *Molecular and cellular biochemistry*, 350, 113-118.

Sala, D., Giachetti, A., & Rosato, A. (2021). Insights into the dynamics of the human zinc transporter ZnT8 by MD simulations. *Journal of chemical information and modeling*, 61(2), 901-912.

Saxena, R., Voight, B. F., Lyssenko, V., Burtt, N. P., de Bakker, P. I., Chen, H., ... & Purcell, S. (2007). Genome-wide association analysis identifies loci for type 2 diabetes and triglyceride levels. *Science*, 316(5829), 1331-1336.

Schulze, M. B., Manson, J. E., Ludwig, D. S., Colditz, G. A., Stampfer, M. J., Willett, W. C., & Hu, F. B. (2004). Sugar-sweetened beverages, weight gain, and incidence of type 2 diabetes in young and middle-aged women. *Jama*, 292(8), 927-934.

Scott, L. J., Bonnycastle, L. L., Willer, C. J., Sprau, A. G., Jackson, A. U., Narisu, N., ... & Boehnke, M. (2006). Association of transcription factor 7-like 2 (TCF7L2) variants with type 2 diabetes in a Finnish sample. *diabetes*, 55(9), 2649-2653.

Scott, L. J., Mohlke, K. L., Bonnycastle, L. L., Willer, C. J., Li, Y., Duren, W. L., ... & Boehnke, M. (2007). A genome-wide association study of type 2 diabetes in Finns detects multiple susceptibility variants. *Science*, 316(5829), 1341-1345.

Shea, J., Agarwala, V., Philippakis, A. A., Maguire, J., Banks, E., DePristo, M., ... & Altshuler, D. (2011). Comparing strategies to fine-map the association of common SNPs at chromosome 9p21 with type 2 diabetes and myocardial infarction. *Nature genetics*, *43*(8), 801-805.

Shu, L., Matveyenko, A. V., Kerr-Conte, J., Cho, J. H., McIntosh, C. H., & Maedler, K. (2009). Decreased TCF7L2 protein levels in type 2 diabetes mellitus correlate with downregulation of GIP-and GLP-1 receptors and impaired beta-cell function. *Human molecular genetics*, *18*(13), 2388-2399.

Skoczek, D., Dulak, J., & Kachamakova-Trojanowska, N. (2021). Maturity onset diabetes of the young - new approaches for disease modelling. *International journal of molecular sciences*, 22(14), 7553.

Sladek, R., Rocheleau, G., Rung, J., Dina, C., Shen, L., Serre, D., ... & Froguel, P. (2007). A genome-wide association study identifies novel risk loci for type 2 diabetes. *Nature*, 445(7130), 881-885.

Sokolova, E. A., Bondar, I. A., Shabelnikova, O. Y., Pyankova, O. V., & Filipenko, M. L. (2015). Replication of KCNJ11 (p. E23K) and ABCC8 (p. S1369A) association in Russian diabetes mellitus 2 type cohort and meta-analysis. *PLoS One*, *10*(5), e0124662.

Song, J., Yang, Y., Mauvais-Jarvis, F., Wang, Y. P., & Niu, T. (2017). KCNJ11, ABCC8 and TCF7L2 polymorphisms and the response to sulfonylurea treatment in patients with type 2 diabetes: a bioinformatics assessment. *BMC medical genetics*, *18*(1), 1-17.

Spielman, R. S., McGinnis, R. E., & Ewens, W. J. (1993). Transmission test for linkage disequilibrium: the insulin gene region and insulin-dependent diabetes mellitus (IDDM). *American journal of human genetics*, 52(3), 506.

Steinthorsdottir, V., Thorleifsson, G., Reynisdottir, I., Benediktsson, R., Jonsdottir, T., Walters, G. B., ... & Stefansson, K. (2007). A variant in CDKAL1 influences insulin response and risk of type 2 diabetes. *Nature genetics*, *39*(6), 770-775.

Takada, I., & Makishima, M. (2020). Peroxisome proliferator-activated receptor agonists and antagonists: A patent review (2014-present). *Expert opinion on therapeutic patents*, *30*(1), 1-13.

The 1000 Genomes Project Consortium (2015). A global reference for human genetic variation. *Nature*, 526(7571), 68.

Tong, Y., Lin, Y., Zhang, Y., Yang, J., Zhang, Y., Liu, H., & Zhang, B. (2009). Association between TCF7L2gene polymorphisms and susceptibility to type 2 diabetes mellitus: a large human genome epidemiology (HuGE) review and meta-analysis. *BMC medical genetics*, *10*(1), 1-25.

Tundo, G. R., Sbardella, D., Ciaccio, C., Grasso, G., Gioia, M., Coletta, A., ... & Coletta, M. (2017). Multiple functions of insulin-degrading enzyme: a metabolic crosslight? *Critical reviews in biochemistry and molecular biology*, 52(5), 554-582.

Turki, A., Al-Zaben, G. S., Khirallah, M., Marmouch, H., Mahjoub, T., & Almawi, W. Y. (2014). Gender-dependent associations of CDKN2A/2B, KCNJ11, POLI, SLC30A8, and TCF7L2 variants with type 2 diabetes in (North African) Tunisian Arabs. *Diabetes Research and Clinical Practice*, *103*(3), e40-e43.

Urakami, T. (2019). Maturity-onset diabetes of the young (MODY): current perspectives on diagnosis and treatment. *Diabetes, metabolic syndrome and obesity: targets and therapy*, 12, 1047.

Vadva, Z., Larsen, C. E., Propp, B. E., Trautwein, M. R., Alford, D. R., & Alper, C. A. (2019). A new pedigree-based SNP haplotype method for genomic polymorphism and genetic studies. *Cells*, *8*(8), 835.

Vallo, J., Arbas, R., Basilio, J. E., Cayabyab, I., Miranda, C. N., Santos, M., ... & Tiongco, R. E. (2022). Association of the Pro12Ala gene polymorphism with treatment response to thiazolidinediones in patients with type 2 diabetes: a meta-analysis. *International Journal of Diabetes in Developing Countries*, 1-8.

Vasseur, F., Helbecque, N., Lobbens, S., Vasseur-Delannoy, V., Dina, C., Clement, K., ... & Froguel, P. (2005). Hypoadiponectinaemia and high risk of type 2 diabetes are associated with adiponectin-encoding (ACDC) gene promoter variants in morbid obesity: evidence for a role of ACDC in diabesity. *Diabetologia*, *48*(5), 892-899.

Villareal, D. T., Koster, J. C., Robertson, H., Akrouh, A., Miyake, K., Bell, G. I., ... & Polonsky, K. S. (2009). Kir6. 2 variant E23K increases ATP-sensitive K+ channel activity and is associated with impaired insulin release and enhanced insulin sensitivity in adults with normal glucose tolerance. *Diabetes*, *58*(8), 1869-1878.

Vionnet, N., Passa, P., & Froguel, P. (1993). Prevalence of mitochondrial gene mutations in families with diabetes mellitus. *The Lancet*, *342*(8884), 1429-1430.

Virendra, S. A., Kumar, A., Chawla, P. A., & Mamidi, N. (2022). Development of Heterocyclic PPAR Ligands for Potential Therapeutic Applications. *Pharmaceutics*, *14*(10), 2139.

Vujkovic, M., Keaton, J. M., Lynch, J. A., Miller, D. R., Zhou, J., Tcheandjieu, C., ... & Saleheen, D. (2020). Discovery of 318 new risk loci for type 2 diabetes and related vascular outcomes among 1.4 million participants in a multi-ancestry meta-analysis. *Nature genetics*, 52(7), 680-691.

Whincup, P. H., Kaye, S. J., Owen, C. G., Huxley, R., Cook, D. G., Anazawa, S., ... & Yarbrough, D. E. (2008). Birth weight and risk of type 2 diabetes: a systematic review. *Jama*, *300*(24), 2886-2897.

Wang, W., Barratt, B. J., Clayton, D. G., & Todd, J. A. (2005). Genome-wide association studies: theoretical and practical concerns. *Nature Reviews Genetics*, 6(2), 109-118.

Warncke, K., Eckert, A., Kapellen, T., Kummer, S., Raile, K., Dunstheimer, D., ... & Holl, R. W. (2022). Clinical presentation and long-term outcome of patients with KCNJ11/ABCC8 variants: Neonatal diabetes or MODY in the DPV registry from Germany and Austria. *Pediatric Diabetes*, 23(7), 999-1008.

Weedon, M. N., McCarthy, M. I., Hitman, G., Walker, M., Groves, C. J., Zeggini, E., ... & Frayling, T. M. (2006). Combining information from common type 2 diabetes risk polymorphisms improves disease prediction. *PLoS medicine*, 3(10), e374.

Welters, H. J., & Kulkarni, R. N. (2008). Wnt signaling: relevance to β-cell biology and diabetes. *Trends in Endocrinology & metabolism*, 19(10), 349-355.

Wheeler, E., & Barroso, I. (2011). Genome-wide association studies and type 2 diabetes. *Briefings in functional genomics*, 10(2), 52-60.

Willemsen, G., Ward, K. J., Bell, C. G., Christensen, K., Bowden, J., Dalgård, C., ... & Spector, T. (2015). The concordance and heritability of type 2 diabetes in 34,166 twin pairs from international twin registers: the discordant twin (DISCOTWIN) consortium. *Twin Research and Human Genetics*, 18(6), 762-771.

Zeggini, E., Weedon, M. N., Lindgren, C. M., Frayling, T. M., Elliott, K. S., Lango, H., ... & Hattersley, A. T. (2007). Replication of genome-wide association signals in UK samples reveals risk loci for type 2 diabetes. *Science*, 316(5829), 1336-1341.

Zhang, C., Qi, L., Hunter, D. J., Meigs, J. B., Manson, J. E., van Dam, R. M., & Hu, F. B. (2006). Variant of transcription factor 7-like 2 (TCF7L2) gene and the risk of type 2 diabetes in large cohorts of US women and men. *Diabetes*, 55(9), 2645-2648.

Zhang, S., Sha, Q., Chen, H. S., Dong, J., & Jiang, R. (2003). Transmission/disequilibrium test based on haplotype sharing for tightly linked markers. *The American Journal of Human Genetics*, 73(3), 566-579.

Zhao, T., Liu, Z., Zhang, D., Liu, Y., Yang, Y., Zhou, D., ... & Xu, H. (2011). The ENPP1 K121Q polymorphism is not associated with type 2 diabetes or obesity in the Chinese Han population. *Journal of human genetics*, 56(1), 12-16.

Zhu, M., & Zhao, S. (2007). Candidate gene identification approach: progress and challenges. *International journal of biological sciences*, 3(7), 420.

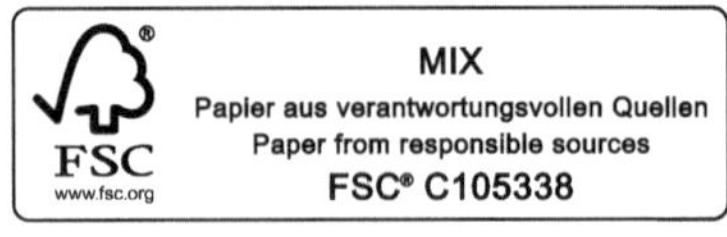

Printed by Books on Demand GmbH, Norderstedt / Germany